Therapeutic Eurythmy for Children

Therapeutic Eurythmy for Children

From Early Childhood to Adolescence

Anne-Maidlin Vogel

SteinerBooks

Translated and edited from the German by Isabel DeAngelis-Suedhof,
Anne Bouwmeester and Terry Boardman.

The back cover poem is by Hedwig Diestel, a twentieth century German poet.

SteinerBooks
www.steinerbooks.org
an imprint of Anthroposophic Press, Inc.
610 Main Street, Suite 1
Great Barrington, MA 01230

Originally published in German as *Heileurythmie für Kinder im ersten und zweiten Jahrsiebt* by (Verlag am Goetheanum, Dornach 2007). Translated and edited by Isabel De Angelis-Suedhof, Anne Bouwmeester and Terry Boardman. Compiled by Norman Francis Vogel and friends.

Copyright 2007 by Norman Francis Vogel

Library of Congress Cataloging-in-Publication data is available.

When the vowels A E I O U are referred to in therapeutic eurythmy exercises in English, they are rendered in this book as follows:

A   as in father
E   as in say
I   as in see
O   as in bowl
U   as in moon
OU   as in thou or how
CH   similar to whistling; like the H in huge or human

The original German poems can be found in the appendices.

— Translator's note

Dedicated to My Beloved Anne-Maidlin

Contents

Introduction

The First Fourteen Years of the Child's Life

Disharmonious Conditions

Appendices

About This Book

ONE MUST NOT LOOK UPON nor use the exercises described in this book as recipes. The human organism has lost its harmonious constitution in our modern times. The life, soul and bodily forces within the patient must be recognized by the therapeutic eurythmist, and then be brought into balance before one begins with the exercises themselves. The therapeutic eurythmist must form a picture for herself as to whether the ill child or adult standing before the therapist is so constituted due to the patient's bodily sheaths having become hardened, or because these sheaths have been shifted (for example: thinking forces pressing down into the feeling life or the other way around, or the will forces shooting up into the feeling or into the head areas, or indeed any combined imbalance). A phenomenon has appeared more and more often over the last twenty years: children and adults have ego forces that are weak or inactive (could this have a connection with artificial insemination or with test-tube babies?). The therapeutic eurythmist must exercise patience and a trained sense of empathy in observing the children or adult patient in order to be able to apply the therapeutic exercises appropriately. Above all he or she must be able to distinguish between examples of the above-mentioned contemporary phenomena and conditions resulting from temperament: **sanguine – nervousness; phlegmatic – apathy; choleric – inactivity, frustration; melancholic – resignation**.

The therapeutic eurythmy training in the 1960s and 70s, in which Anne-Maidlin was a student, took place in Dornach, Switzerland and in Vienna, Austria. The two leading teachers were Trude Thetter and Ilse Rolofs. The depth of perception and the many years of experience of these two teachers helped to give Anne-Maidlin the tools from which she was able to forge her own individual and intuitive way. Her love and joy for all her patients, especially children, made her a very sought-after therapeutic eurythmist in America, Austria and England where she was active for over thirty years. Her co-workers, students and patients relate that when she entered a room, peace and joy filled it. She gave all of herself to help all those who came into contact with her and she was loved by everyone!

This collection touches only a small section of Anne-Maidlin's therapeutic work. The main part of it cannot be expressed in words or forms. It was her rich spirit-soul filled with joy and light which set the healing process in motion the moment a patient entered the room. This happened before a word was spoken or an exercise begun!

Anne-Maidlin's soul-spirit quietly, strongly, accompanies what appears on the following pages. It is hoped that those who study this workbook, even those she never met, can feel a small spark of her real being from time to time.

Preface

IT WAS A PLEASURE TO BE ASKED by Norman Francis Vogel to write a preface to Anne-Maidlin Vogel's life work *Therapeutic Eurythmy for Children*. Firstly because as a pediatrician I know how effectively eurythmy therapy as a movement therapy can be in treating physical and mental developmental disorders, and secondly because it was always something special to meet Anne-Maidlin Vogel at the council meetings of heads of eurythmy therapy training centers held in the Medical Section at the Goetheanum. Apart from the work that needed to be done for the council meetings, and the effort involved in international collaboration on quality criteria, one could always sense her very genuine interest and pleasure in meeting with colleagues. You found yourself immediately in deep conversation and a sharing of personal views and experiences.

It was all the more of a shock, then, when her life ended unexpectedly at the age of 59 due to serious illness, calling her away at the very zenith of her work. And so we also cannot appreciate it highly enough that over the last seven years, following his wife's death, Norman Vogel made every possible effort to organize her material and documents relating to training and practice, and determine what would be suitable for passing on to her professional colleagues. The result is a rich work for professional practice that can be warmly recommended to any eurythmy therapist, physician and also teacher working with children and teenagers. They will find not only a treasury of examples for possible exercises but also many useful and valuable references to personal development and further training for therapists.

The eurythmy therapy exercises with premature infants, babies and young children up to the age of four are most precious, for not much has yet been published for this age group. The quotes from anthroposophic physicians and experienced eurythmy therapists included in the book assume that the reader is familiar with the anthroposophic view of the human being and its terminology. However, even interested lay people will be able to follow many descriptions and sketches of individual exercises, for it is all based on the healthy movement patterns of the developing organism. Study of the speech-eurythmy exercises in particular, or specific speech sounds and sequences of these used, for instance, for postural problems, enuresis or lack of concentration, can encourage the reader to study the laws of eurythmy and eurythmy therapy as speech, music, rhythm, gesture and posture transformed into movement.

I hope this book on eurythmy therapy, at last available, will help to close a long-standing gap in the field of pediatrics and the work of school doctors.

MICHAELA GLÖCKLER, MD
Head of the Medical Section, Dornach, Switzerland
Dornach, January 2007

Introduction

Guidelines for Therapeutic Eurythmists

(Ilse Rolofs)

Three main requirements Rudolf Steiner made for teachers:

1. Enliven yourself with the capacity of fantasy!

2. Have the courage for truth!

3. Sharpen your senses for an inner responsibility of heart!

Mrs. Rolofs' brother, a priest, received these words from Dr. Steiner:

"Polarities must always work together in the world. For example, medical doctors, priests and teachers working together would mean that each one gives actively of himself or herself without disturbing the sphere of the other(s)."

General Practical Indications

(Ilse Rolofs)

* Take children for therapeutic eurythmy lessons four days a week: Monday, Tuesday, Wednesday, and Friday. Take the teachers on Thursday. They also are much in need of therapeutic eurythmy and Thursday is the day for their meeting as well.

* The time for each child: 10–15 minutes

* Take part in the presentation of each pupil on admission to first grade.

* When possible take part in all conferences pertaining to these children. The school doctor should as well! Nurture a good state of working together with the eurythmy teachers.

* About fetching the children:
    – The very first time you yourself should take the children out of their lesson.
    – Then the children should go to get one another.
    – Take the same child always at the same time. When the child is being taken out of his lesson, try to make as little disturbance as possible.
    – Inform the teacher early enough.

* Have the child's desk-neighbor fill him in on what he missed while he was at the therapeutic eurythmy lesson. This can be done in the break.

* Leave their shoes in front of the door (even their own karma stays in front of the door, and my own too). The children should have their eurythmy shoes in their desks so that no confusion comes about.

* The therapeutic eurythmy room should always be nicely kept up; there should always be flowers. The therapeutic eurythmist too should be clean and tidy (no stains, no ripped hems). Children want their teacher to be immaculate.

* Do not leave your shoes or things lying around in the therapeutic eurythmy room. Above all you must never give the appearance of being exhausted, rather you must always radiate a calmness and peacefulness. Take care to make sure that your own

clothes are well color-coordinated. The children have to look at your clothing the whole time! The children must have the feeling that the therapeutic eurythmist can bring everything into order (heal all). One should know a bit about First Aid and have a small First Aid kit handy.

* The period of time between Christmas and Easter is often longer than seven weeks. Therefore one can use these surplus weeks to get to know the children better by sitting in on the lessons.

* Continuously train your insight into seeing that which lives spiritually within the child. In the evening think about each child and try to imagine how he would look if he were healthy.

* With a great sense of respect for the child, try to enter into his inharmonious movements: how does he feel because he moves thus. This is the starting point to try to find the appropriate therapy. One must guide the child in such a way that he comes to the point in which he truly overcomes his unhealthiness.

* Rudolf Steiner emphasizes the importance that eurythmists always wear something on their heads, in summer and in winter, and that they wear a girdle to avoid problems of descending abdominal organs, and that they use heel pads (approximately 1/2 inch) in their shoes.

* Eurythmists should work three-quarters of the year and have a vacation the other quarter of the year. Also, one should rest in loose-fitting clothing for two hours during the noon break. Not necessarily sleeping, but resting. After the birth of your child you should have a break for three years until the child says "I."

* One should seek new impulses for therapeutic eurythmy from Rudolf Steiner's lectures (Lectures to the Physicians or to the Workers, etc.). Try to connect your own strength and powers to that which is the light of knowledge of the world or out of Anthroposophy itself.

* Take on little social jobs within the school: Christmas cards, colleagues' birthdays.

* Therapeutic eurythmists should teach no more than 12 hours of eurythmy a week, but can teach other subjects to complete a full teaching schedule, to a maximum of 18 hours, according to Ilse Rolofs.

* Every individual has his own state of true health. Obstacles must simply be removed in order to unfold it. Don't make the child healthy too soon, he needs his own time to come to terms with his proper state of health.

* When you take on new children come to know them by how they make a circle, a pentagon, how they form an A, how they walk and move and what their handwriting is like. Include their angel!

* If a child doesn't have a particular virtue (for example, he has no courage and must learn this) then you should practise this soul mood in eurythmy. Help the children to truly overcome themselves!

* Keep strictly to the time. Try to take the younger children up until 12:00 noon, as long as the sun is still ascending. The older children (Upper School) you can take after 12:00.

* After seven weeks have a little therapeutic eurythmy festival and a talk with the child's main teacher.

* A four-term year is recommended:
  a) September–Christmas (Christmas vacation)
  b) Christmas–14 days before Easter (the last two weeks she doesn't give any lessons; she sits in on the children's lessons)
  c) Easter–May
  d) May–July

* Ilse Rolofs had groups. Usually 80 children per day. She worked five hours a day. Individual children (difficult cases and restless ones) she took during the main lesson.

Fundamental Exercises

1. Begin the therapeutic eurythmy lesson with

    I A O
or T A O
or T L M

End the lesson with either:

a) Love – E

b) A – Veneration

c) any other soul-exercise

The main therapeutic eurythmy exercise you would do in-between.

2. Stepping rhythms to the following text, slowly getting faster, and quickly getting slower

The old maid goose, she looked and saw what others do
Thought I can too, and then began to dance, Ah!
Oh old maid goose, oh let it be,
You'll only break your back and knee.
The goose tripped over a stone and rolled
She broke her leg, it ended so, the dancing.
So must it be my old maid goose, the dance is not for everyone;
So leave it to the others.

(With older children, one can also speak the text, or step it while speaking.)

3. *Stepping rhythms and clapping* (Ilse Rolofs)

Morning: short-long-short / short-long-short (while walking and clapping)

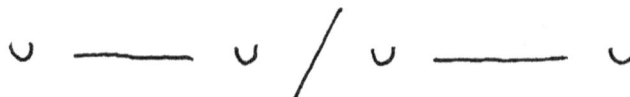

$$\cup \quad \text{——} \quad \cup \; / \; \cup \quad \text{——} \quad \cup$$

In therapeutic eurythmy one should slowly get faster and quickly get slower. *(Ilse Rolofs)*

Evening: long-short-long / long-short-long (while walking and clapping)

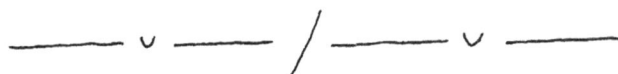

$$\text{——} \; \cup \; \text{——} \; / \; \text{——} \; \cup \; \text{——}$$

4. *The archetype of walking* (from Lory Maier-Smits)

Three-fold walking: Standing on the balls of both feet with one leg slightly in front of the other as if taking a step. One lifts oneself onto the tips of the toes, shifts the weight from the back foot to the foot in front which is then lowered onto the ground. At the same time there is a similar movement to that of the R gesture going through the soles of the feet and even through the entire body. The back foot is carefully being carried through the air and then with only the tip of the toe is placed onto the floor. Once again there follows this R-type of movement: one goes onto the tips of the toes of both feet, the entire body's weight shifts from the back foot onto that of the front foot. Meanwhile, the back foot frees itself and is carried carefully through the air while the other foot is being lowered from the tip of the toe onto the entire foot. Once again the foot which is carefully being carried through the air is being placed with only the tip of the toe onto the floor and this R, a type of rolling, shifting of weight – a kind of expansion throughout the entire body, and then one starts all over again. While carrying the foot (close to the floor), one's stature is relaxed (like in an M gesture where the posture is almost like in a slight contraction). In the moment that one is standing on the tips of the toes of both feet and one shifts the weight from the back onto the front foot, the body is in a more expanding posture.

5. *Circles*

The circle stands for calmness, self-assurance and a feeling of self-containment.

*The First Fourteen Years
of the Child's Life*

I. Therapeutic Eurythmy for Babies

"One should not let a child that hasn't turned three do eurythmy because the spiritual forces are still working to build up his physical body. **In therapeutic eurythmy this is not the case.** If there are signs of abnormalities: the child cannot lift itself up, squinting, deformation of the head, etc., then you may start with therapeutic eurythmy exercises quite early but only in a proper child-like manner."

—Margarete Kirchner-Bockholt, *Fundamental Principles of Curative Eurythmy*, p. 28

1. Do many exercises with a small-sized veil and different sounds:

a) Place veil material over both arms and move like V.

b) Take the veil material in your hand and let it fly like the wind.

c) With veil material in hands, turn like a wheel (R). Do all the consonants as if with an object, only the object is a small-sized veil.

d) Roll the veil material into a ball in one hand, both hands like a B around the veil like a bud, then slowly open your hands. The veil opens up like a flower (A).

e) Lay the veil material on your arm with an enclosing gesture B (I enclose the child with my veiled arm or he places his veiled arm around me).

f) Veil over your head: F blowing so that the veil flies or hold the piece of veil at a corner and the rest of the veil roll up in your hand, then with an F push it forwards sending it out into the room.

Sophia Hablützel, a therapeutic eurythmist, says never to do an L with small children, nor for 1st and 2nd graders. It excarnates and the children must incarnate.

Always lead the children in a circle going to the left: the direction of the etheric. Guide them into the etheric.

2. Exercises for those born prematurely

Incarnating sequence (for example   A O U E)

Evolutionary sequence: B M D N R L G CH F S H T

- Form large gestures while standing at a distance
- Go closer and make the gestures somewhat smaller
- Go even closer and make the gestures even smaller
- Then form very small, gentle gestures over the child
  (repeating the entire sequence each time!)

3. Different Sounds

A is the sound for early childhood. Often it is the first sound that the child speaks. It helps the process of incarnation because the movement of reaching out in two directions in space in the A gesture has as its opposite movement a streaming in, a flowing inwards of the spiritual (incarnation). A and E lead into the incarnating process, O marks the beginning of the excarnating process. B is the consonant for little children.

4. U with the arms

Place the baby on your lap and rock to the right and left rhythmically (4 x 4) while speaking the four lines. With "Cuckoo" lift the baby up doing U with the arms. One can do this to help against rickets.

Tick, tock, tick, tock
I'm a little cuckoo clock
Tick, tock, tick, tock
Now I'm striking one o'clock (two o'clock, three o'clock, etc.)
Cuckoo ... Cuckoo (as often as the clock strikes: at 4 o'clock = 4 x Cuckoo)

5. U *(with the feet and B)*

Place the baby on your lap in such a way that he can push his feet against your stomach.

While speaking the first line, tap the baby's right foot with your palm. With the second line, tap his left foot. Speaking the third line, guide his feet into an U, and with the fourth line make a B gesture around the baby.

Shoe the little horse
Shoe the little mare
But let the little coltie ride
Bare, bare, bare.

6. Exercises for falling asleep *(from Angela Rascher, a therapeutic eurythmist)*

Hold the baby in your arms while walking backwards and open your wings into the back-space in A (etherically). Then walk forwards with the feeling of O around the child. (Only experience the O etherically since obviously you can't make a physical gesture with the child in your arms!) Do this only 3 times and end going backwards with the A again, as in the beginning.

7. B *(before going to sleep)*

The sound B survives all troubles and fears. (from Hebrew). The most beautiful B is visible in the Sistine Madonna. Dr. Steiner indicated to have restless children look at a picture of The Sistine Madonna before they go to bed and at the same time gently stroke the child's head. (this gives a protection for a child's missing sheltering-sheath).

Light and warmth
From the holy Spirits of the World
Enclose me.   (to this only a single B gesture)

II. The First Seven Years

"If you place demands on how a child should be, nobody can define that. One must toil through difficult studies in order to psychologically understand how a child really is: a learning to understand the child, not to think that they must be a certain way."

—Rudolf Steiner

General Exercises

1. Introducing L

Clap your hands from below upwards then continue going outwards after each clap, like a blossoming, or like: "blowing raindrops."

2. Introducing A – H

A : with your hands (as in piety) like a caterpillar that eats and becomes fatter and fatter which then flies away as a butterfly.

H: From my heart into my hands
   I feel the breath of God

—R. Steiner
(See Appendices p. 195 for original German and complete English versions.)

3. Exercise for incarnating

long-long-short-long-long; long-long-short-long-long

a) Standing with feet separated, one slightly in front of the other: Rock forwards on the first long bending into your knee. Rock backwards into the second long. Then make a short step forwards, on the short. With the next long go forwards once again, rocking into your bent knee. Go backwards on the long. Then go forwards with the next long rocking into your knee. The next long going backwards and then the short once again with a step forwards.

b) Do the same as above but begin rocking backwards and therefore do the short step backwards.

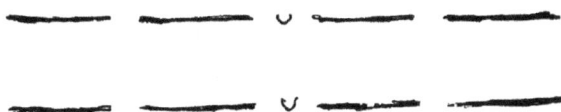

4. From "We" to "I"

− The child and the therapist hold hands and move in a circle - the feeling of "We"
− The child and the therapist stand opposite one another, touching each other's hands in a D − the feeling of "You"
− The child touches his own self − the feeling of "I"

5. Rod exercise for incarnating

Place two or four copper rods in the form of a cross.

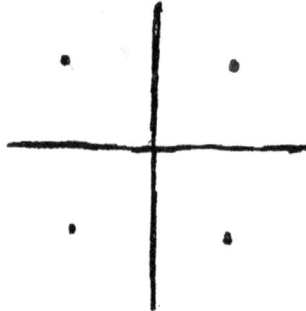

The child should jump in an U into every square formed by the cross.

6. Hope U soul gesture *(Marianne Johnson, a therapeutic eurythmist, used this imagination)*

How shall we show this to the child?

The gesture of "Hope"
as a large bowl filled with bird food.

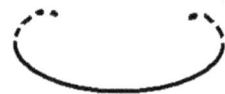

The birds fly from above downwards into the bowl
and peck at the bird food.
With the raising of your toes the little birds are being called.

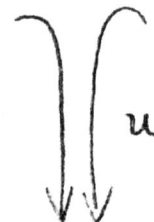

7. Exercises for agility

With your feet toe to heel, while climbing up a vertically held copper rod with your hands.

One could alter this by having your feet move twice as fast as your hands, or just the opposite.

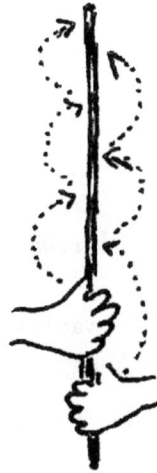

8. Vowels with the rod

A little poem for the vowels:

Be a shining star above me.	A
Be an angel to protect me.	E
Be a guiding light to lead me.	I
Be a rose of love within me.	O
Be the beauty shining through me.	U

Exercises to Strengthen the Etheric
from A.-M. Vogel

1. A E I O U
(Do all the vowels with a child: sitting or kneeling on a stool while singing)

a) Large gestures, forwards (musical scale upwards) Large gestures, downwards (musical scale descending)

b) Form vowels from elbows to fingers (half an arm)

c) With hands (Angels' sounds)

d) With fingers (butterfly sounds) (Four is the number of incarnation: do gestures from large to small to help the child to incarnate.)

2. A E I O U *(in walking)*

In his second lecture on therapeutic eurythmy, Rudolf Steiner says:

"One can take all the movements which we have now described and thus increase the effect by doing them while stepping. And you would achieve especially a lot for a weak child when, for example, you instruct him to do an A gesture while walking just as we have done now."

3. A E I O U *(on in-winding spirals)*

"In-winding spirals strengthen the etheric." —Rudolf Steiner

4. *Changing speeds*

Slowly becoming fast, quickly becoming slow

Text: (walking, running, jumping)

"We ride so swiftly through field and woods,
The mountains both down and up.
And if someone falls right off his horse,
He falls very softly and picks himself up.
The way goes over stones and slime,
We give the horse the reins to lead,
And ride in the bright sunshine,
So fast like wings for speed.
Hey Ha over stones and slime
Hey Ha and into the stall – Yah!"

—Traditional (See Appendices p. 195 for original German.)

5. *Forms* (alternating between straight lines and curves)

6. *Contrasts/Opposites*

a) "Oh how slowly   high-low   big-little
    oh how slowly   fast-slow   running-walking
    moves the snail   light-heavy   straight-curved
    from spot to spot..."   quiet-loud

b) _____   Place seven rods on the floor:
    _____   Play the melody of the pentatonic scale
    _____   descending while running or jumping over the seven rods
    _____   e d b a g e d – "listening" with the toes

c) Play a melody of fifths, as follows:

A is the center tone

A-E the inner-heart region

A-D the lower region

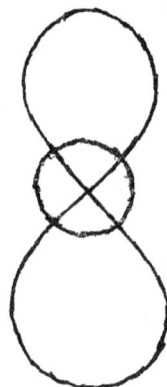

d) Little horsey (Have the children ride, then stand still)

"Little horsey hop hop hop, little horsey stop stop stop."

e) Heel-toe as contrast

The left foot begins with the toes, then goes to the heel;
the right foot begins with the heel, then goes to the toes.

Fiddler Hans, fiddle once
our daughter dances
she has a colored skirt on
Oh my, and how she prances.   (vowels on the poem)

f) With your heels hammer like the dwarves; walk very quietly on tip-toes so that they
   don't wake up Snow White.

g) Veneration-A (Soul Gesture)

Make an A eurythmically with your arms in front of you and above your head, then instead of going into a eurythmical H, as is often done, do a warm L with the shoulders over the back. This brings the A more into the body, thus incarnating.

h.) Place rods on the floor:

"Jack be nimble,   Jack be quick

(right foot over one rod and back)   (left foot over one rod and back)

Jack jump over,   the candlestick."

(right foot over one rod and back)   (jump over both rods with both feet)

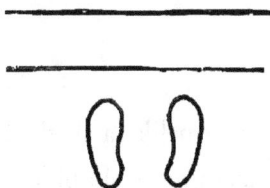

The same exercise can be done to:

Himpelley and Pimpelley make a jump
Himpelley and Pimpelley make a plump! (jump into the knees)

Up into the cherry tree
Who should climb but little me
Hand over hand, then with both hands
Looked out and saw both sea and sands.
Then I jumped from branch to branch
Looked out again, saw a Texas ranch
Ha ha I laughed, and lost my grip   (on laughed, rod falls)
And down I fell in one quick zip!   (crouch down)
Mother came and picked me up
And in her arms went home to sup.   (with B)

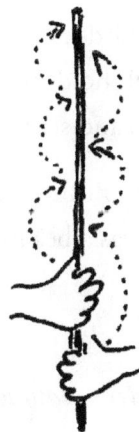

— Inspired by R. L. Stevenson

Exercises for Fearful and TV-Damaged Children

1. U against Fear

A child who is fearful can be strengthened with U. Strengthen him with U, but do not jump. Instead lead his hands together so that he feels his own physical self. Have him place his feet next to each other closely in U with his knees and thighs against one another so that he feels his own body.

Then in walking: one step forwards, bring the other foot decisively in from the side and place it next to the first foot and bend into your knees.

2. The strengthening B

The child makes a good B with one arm like a shield for protection and with the other arm an I above the therapeutic eurythmist's shoulder. The therapeutic eurythmist also makes a B (shield) over the child's shoulder and while doing so, they both look each other in the eyes. This gives courage and strength.

3. The Interval of the Fifth from above downwards

The child does the eurythmical gesture for the interval of the fifth while standing on a footstool, holds this gesture of the fifth, steps down from the stool, releases the gesture in the arms and stands in the prime.

"Sleeping Beauty was a beautiful child, a beautiful child, a beautiful child, Sleeping Beauty was a beautiful child, a beautiful child."   (Fifth)

4. Children damaged by watching television

Dr. Hablützel recommended the above three exercises (Hope-U, strengthening B, and the fifth) for children damaged by watching television. The nerve-sense pole has the upper hand with such children. That's why one should enliven the metabolic and rhythmic poles. Do many walking exercises in order to help achieve "speaking feet." Small steps: dwarf steps, large steps: giant steps while lifting the leg and foot up well and really bringing them down again breathing out into the earth. Here comes the giant gigantically big, the steps are also gigantically big.

In order to enliven the metabolic or the rhythmic system: if the developmental process is damaged, then do the "Evolutionary Sequence" in that damaged zone. Sometimes take only parts of the "Evolutionary Sequence." Repeat the consonants over and over again.

5. Recommended medicaments for such children

Dr. Hablützel had them given a light massage with cassisis oil and then rolled them up in a pre-warmed linen cloth for half an hour in order to activate the metabolic and rhythmic systems, to create a sheath of warmth. He also prescribed silver as a medicament.

Exercises for Very-Sensitive Children

They do not want to put their feet on the ground.

Do B and B M D perhaps standing behind the child as well.

When the speech development is disturbed: (this was the case with one particular child) the vowels help to bring about the forming of the consonants in the front part of the mouth. (Rudolf Steiner, *Curative Eurythmy Course,* lecture 2. Vowels)

Make the gestures for all the vowels and consonants so strongly for the child that he wants to imitate them. The small child doesn't always need to do everything himself but rather he should experience in his own soul-spiritual space that which we eurythmically do around him.

1. To strengthen the ability to imitate

A E I   I E A

A   has within it the forces of imitation.

Exercises to Help Children to Incarnate

1. Little mice game

"They scribble and scrabble along the floor,
They squeeze and squeak beneath the door,
They run, they dance, they turn about
And hush, appear within the house."

2. Kiebitz

"Good horsey I do give you shoes
Be brave and true like stars above
For only then your Lord shall come
And ride with you into the sun,
And ride with you into the sun."

— F. Rückert (Appendices p. 196)

– Roll your feet over the rod
– Roll your feet over the copper ball (so that the feet can grip better)
– R with the legs: let the little horsey scrape with his hoof while I say R (can be used for both above examples)

3. Hexameter *(tapping on the sole of the foot)*

4 – the number for incarnation

"Shoemaker, shoemaker make me some shoes
Brown leather, fine leather, I come to choose."

4. A-U: with the hands and the whole arm

"Sleep in peace, butterfly you,   (A and U in the hands, with the arms and
Close your wings, slowly do.   also with the legs, as grandfather butterfly)
Open, A; close, oo;
Open, A; close, oo;
Keep quite still, keep quite still.
Ah, butterfly you."

5. Toes E and heels; A-E in the arms

Change quickly toe to heal, back and forth

"Fiddler Hans, fiddle once ...
Our daughter dances,   (A – E)
She has a colored dress on
Oh my, and how she prances."   (A – E)

6. Toes to heels plus E with the feet

"Flashing fish jumping fish
happy in the waves that swish"

7. U against fears

U ("oo") against fears: step forwards, bring the other leg sidewards next to the first; almost
hitting against it.

8. Rolling the feet over the rod

"Ri ra roach, we're riding in the coach   (one coach swinging further)
We're riding in a tortoise shell   (two "coaches"...)
A penny rings the bell so well   (three "coaches" in the circle)
Ri ra roach, we're riding in the coach."

9. Place the rod on the floor *(similar to exercise on p. 31)*

right foot over one rod and back   "Jack be nimble
left foot over one rod and back   Jack be quick

right foot over one rod and back   Jack jump over
then jump over the rod with I "ee"   the candle stick."

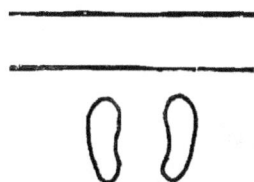

10. Three-part walking

"Something wanders across the field
It's wearing a black & white dress
And has a pair of stockings red
Going a-clipperty, clap, clap, clap
Going a-clipperty, clap clap, clap
The frogs begin to schlap, schlap, schlap
Who can tell what's happening?"

11. Rolling the rod up and down your arms

"Oh how the beech tree sways in the wind
Rocking the little bullfinch child so dear
The last one, the dearest high up in the tree
That chirps so softly like in a dream"

(fingers on top of and underneath the rod like "qui qui")

This exercise may also be used for relationship to others and to the surrounding world. Do it in pairs: one rod between each other, another rod placed on the floor.

III. Children in Their Ninth Year

From Dr. Joop von Dam:

"Between the ninth and tenth year of a child's life is an important moment in the child's development, especially in the warmth organization of the human being. The "I" or Ego of the human being draws into the metabolic-limb system. The rhythm between breathing and the circulation of the blood (pulse) become 1:4 (for each person slightly different). At this time the child begins to run from his legs instead of being steered by his head like a doll. They leave their childhood Paradise. In this period of time they can have headaches, stomach aches, back and shoulder pains and become quite ill as well."

General Exercises

I A O   (harmonizing)

D T   (to help bring warmth into the digestive system)

G L M

1. Alliterations

a) from *Beowulf*

"Forth from the fence   Came over clouds
of the misty moorlands   Until he saw clearly
Grendel came gliding   glittering with gold plates
Gods wrath he bore.   The mead hall of men."

b) "Peter, Peter, pumpkin eater
   had a wife and couldn't keep her
   Put her in a pumpkin shell
 There he kept her very well."

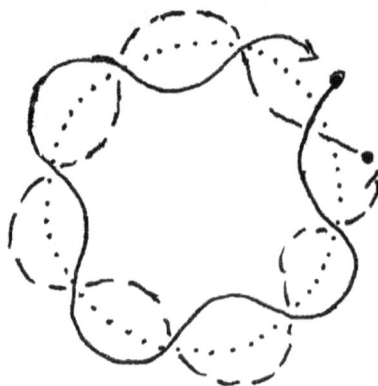

(Weaving around in a circle in and out with two groups in two directions and clapping the hands of the 2nd group coming towards you on the right, the left, and then alternating)

2. Agility-E (with variations for the arms)

Very fast and graceful, alternating between hitting with your heel on your knee and softly and gracefully with your toes on the floor.

3. Jumping over rods

a)

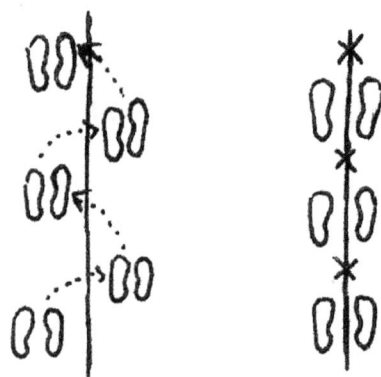

b) E placing a coin or a seashell at the crossing point; walking or jumping over forwards)

Within and around the ninth year of a child's life, the children need special exercises for their legs and feet which go beyond the rhythmical and are more than just moving along forms. The left leg lives in the rising bloodstream. It has the striving force, the inner warmth that one soulfully and wilfully expresses in steadfastness. It is musically lighter than the right leg. It is the leg used for the upbeat. The right leg experiences the in-drawing circulation of the blood; the direction towards the physical. The right leg feels more the outer supporting force which gives us a sense of security in our soul and will spheres. Musically seen, the I or Ego lies in the right side being the heavier part of the beat. In the third lecture of *Psychology of Body, Soul and Spirit* (Anthroposophic Press, Hudson, 1999) Rudolf Steiner says that from left to right we go into the physical; from right to left we go into the etheric. In walking we always have a feeling of a slight swaying to and fro between the physical and the etheric, between a descending and a rising, buoyant experience.

> Left: steadfastness
> Right: certainty
> —Rosemarie Bock, a therapeutic eurythmist

4. "Staircase exercise" – E

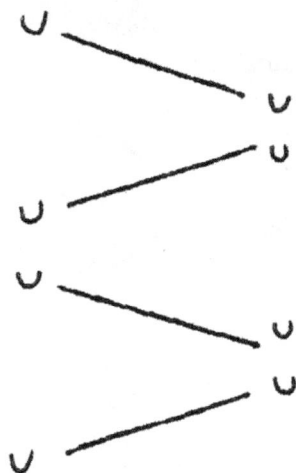

Arms: a large E in front

E above your head

E behind your back

E in front downwards

5. "Big E vowel exercise"

6. Copper ball exercises: *(with a lemniscate form)*

For example to "At the Ringing of the Bells":

To wonder at beauty
Stand guard over truth
Look up to the noble
Resolve on the good
This leadeth man truly
To purpose in living
To right in his doing
To peace in his feeling
To light in his thinking
And teaches him trust
In the workings of God
In all that there is
In the widths of the world
In the depths of the soul.

—Rudolf Steiner (see Appendices p. 196 for original German)

7. "Frère Jacques" (Brother John) exercise: *(also vowels with feet)*

   A   I   A   I   O   O
"Are you sleeping, are you sleeping, brother John, brother John?

   O   I   O   I
Morning bells are ringing, morning bells are ringing:

   I   O   I   O
Ding ding dong, ding ding dong."

8. Hand and feet, foot and hands

(Speaking)	(Do with partner)
Hand	Clap once
And	Drop head down
Two Feet	Jump twice
Foot	Jump once
And	Head up
Two Hands	Clap twice

Then repeat along the circle swinging over to a new partner.

9. Poem for general strengthening

(from Friedl Thomas, eurythmist in Dornach in Rudolf Steiner's time)

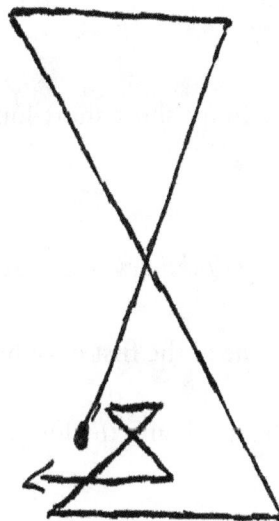

I keep you away, I keep you away,
I help myself.

10. E Exercise in all variations, also Agility-E in all variations

From therapeutic eurythmist Ellen von Dam

Mister East gave a feast
Mister West did his best
Mister North laid the cloth
Mister South burned his mouth
Eating hot potatoes

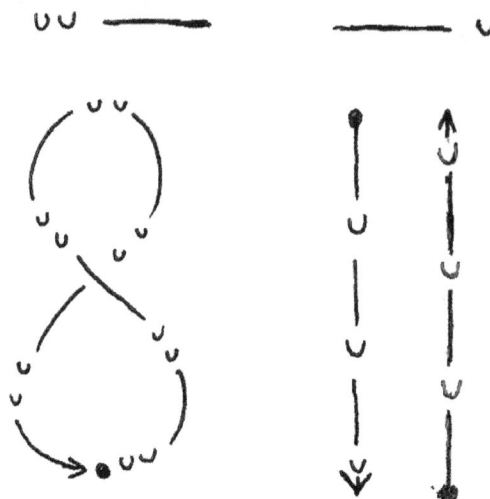

Mister East, etc.   Eating hot potatoes

11. Changing rhythms

Going without a pause from "short-short-long" to "long-short" strengthens the etheric.

12. Rhythm measuring *(Taktieren – long-short   short-short-long)*

From Ilona Schubert, one of the first eurythmists in Dornach

The shorts measure the width and the longs measure the length of the body.

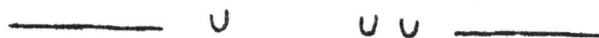

13. Clapping

a) It can have an awakening, lively effect, the child can touch himself/herself and through hearing grasp himself/herself. It may not become too monotone or too mechanical, otherwise the child will begin to hit him/herself and thereby harden his/her movements and his/her listening ability would become dulled.

b) Alternate between clapping with the tips of your fingers, the palms of your hands, your knees, your toes, and the soles of your feet.

c) The clapping should be like the sounding of a gong: resounding on and on, not like catching flies!

d) Clapping with your feet: while jumping up into the air bring your feet together.

14. Stamping *(not into the ground, but rather on the balls of the feet for alliterations)*

15. Reviewing in backward order

(Do not do this with children before they are age 9)

This strengthens the memory.

"By going backwards and retracing the way to their original point of departure, the children will become strengthened in their own experience of themselves (of their own "I" or "Self").

a) Forms - walk forwards and backwards

b) Poems - line for line, forwards and backwards

c) "I" or Ego Line ("ich")

d) "Here I am" (I I A), with all variations

e) Pedagogical (I A O) slowly getting faster, then from very quick, slowly getting very slow.

16. In Speech Formation for 4th-6th grade

———— ∪   ∪ ————

long short   short long

"Steadfast   I stand"   (left leg to the left
                                and somewhat forward)
"Certain   I go"   (right leg to the right
                                and somewhat forward)
"On the earth, through the world."   (jump, bringing the legs together)

The above exercise was inspired by the following verse:

(The feeling of devotion)

Steadfast I stand in existence   (Left foot forward and to the left)
With certainty I tread the path of life   (Right foot forward and to the right)
Love I cherish in the kernel of my being   (Left arm out, shoulder-height)
Hope I plant in every deed.   (Right arm out, shoulder height)
Confidence I place in all my thinking   (Hold positions, feel the pentagram)
These five guide me to my aim,   (Left arm crossing over chest)
These five give me my existence .   (Right arm crossing over chest)

—Rudolf Steiner (See Appendices p. 197 for original German)

IV. Children in Their Twelfth Year

In the twelfth year of life the soul-spiritual widens itself out into the bones. Children in this age often suffer from the vertebrae rubbing against one another (as in Schuermann's disease), as well as problems in the arch of the foot. The inner impulse is often missing which is often neglected by the attitude of the adults as well. The outer carriage is the image of the inner attitude and the children fall much too early into heaviness. At this time one can prevent and help before worse defects arise. By the age of twelve, at the latest, valgus deformities (genu valgum= knock knee or X-legs and genu varum= bow legs) appear. One meets this in boys who tend to be overly-phlegmatic, corpulent, and who don't like to move much. In a certain sense they try to seek protection behind their layers of fat. They don't really want to enter into puberty and so they remain somewhat infantile. Often poor eating habits exist. Also valgus deformities sometimes show themselves (which one discovers when one asks) in that the boy's testicles have not yet descended. With girls one experiences more the illness of anorexia. They also don't want to enter into puberty and unconsciously deny the descent into the lower bodily processes.

Exercises for Defects in Posture
(Ilse Rolofs)

1. G S *(to strengthen the ability to make decisions)*

G – truly free oneself from something dark and inwardly become full of light, having complete control over it; then form an S.

(Don't bring it into an end position with children. With adults bring it into an end position or into the gesture for Scorpion [Scorpio].)

2. *L L L M*

L – lift somewhat slightly over the horizontal zone, 3 times and then guide it into M.

L – from out of the left-right or horizontal balance leading into the vertical uprightness.

3. *Scoliosis L*

3 times: L right; L left, U forwards, A backwards, a quiet S (that is a tender and delicate S) downwards. (from Ilse Rolofs)

4. *C C C D*

For children with problems with their feet. (Children with fallen arches should do a counter growing movement with the D. This is done by going upwards onto the tips of the toes very slowly while performing the D with the arms.

5. *W in relation to vowels*

(The German W, or English V, is the only sound not given by Rudolf Steiner for therapeutic eurythmy.)

V A
V E
V I
V O
V U

 a) forwards
b) backwards
c) begin with vowels (U V, O V...)

6. S R L M sounds of the four elements *(for "enkindling" the children)*

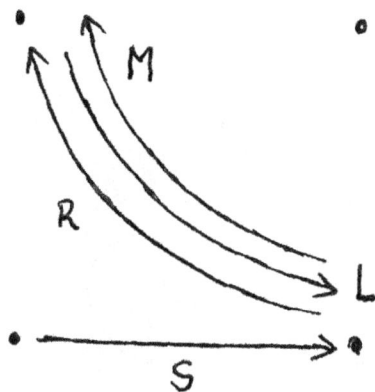

S	R
Fire	**Air**
Will	Courage

L	M
Water	**Earth**
Feeling	Thought
Sensitivity	

Above all one can work with the Rhythmical R, with the airy, refreshing, and cleansing and thereby get rid of the thick and tense atmosphere to a certain degree.

This same exercise was also given to an epileptic girl. It uses sounds that help to further the I or Ego-Organism.

Do the M standing! This can be used in alternation with R L S O on a similar form.

7. Trochee with different vowels; if necessary

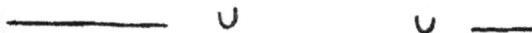

on long, free stepping; on short, the vowel with one step

8. Kiebitz step

9. T A O

10. Exercises for girls with anorexia

a) I A O eventually bending into the knees with A

b) M while walking, (the lower half of legs does M)

c) T L M consonant-related I A O:

d) T U B A

e) B

f) In-winding Spiral   with A – E

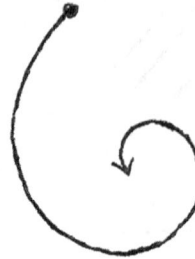

g) Yes – no enhances a deep and free breathing.

11. Exercise for headaches (Ilse Rolofs)

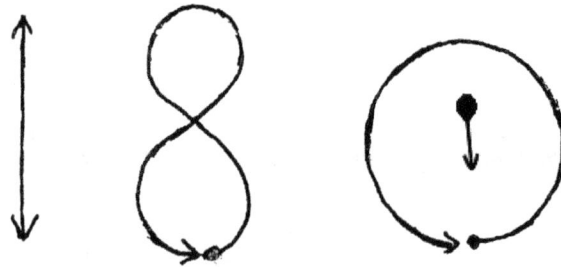

I – You – He
    with vowels

With the HE form, one moves from the middle to the
periphery, with the feeling of devotion, moving around a
Spiritual Being who is in the center. The eurythmist
always faces the center. (given verbally by Rudolf Steiner to
a eurythmist)

12. Different lemniscate exercises

In them the S form is as beautifully found as we also find again in our spine! :

a) Lemniscates that have the direction of front and back:

Affinity   –   Distance
Yes   –   No
Sympathy –   Antipathy

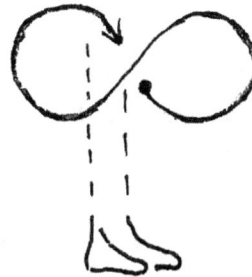

Soul forces, which certainly play a part in back problems.

Now we raise the lemniscate
into the vertical and thus have
the direction of up and down as well.

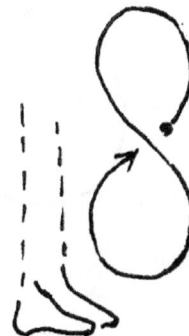

b)

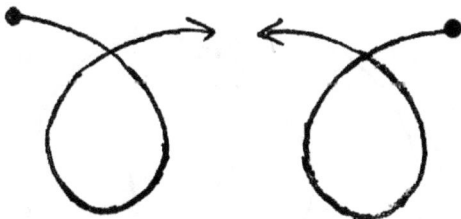

An attempt to put into movement the
feeling of the lecture from Rudolf
Steiner *Die wissenschaft vom Werden des
menschen,* GA 183 (these two forms and
the two forms on the following page)

The spiritual-soul element
of the human being
pushes out into the spiritual-soul
element of the environment
and pushes inwards
against his sub-consciousness.

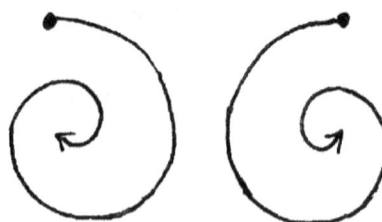

See previous two forms and two forms above. —Rudolf Steiner, *Die Wissenshaft vom Werden des Menschen,* GA 183.

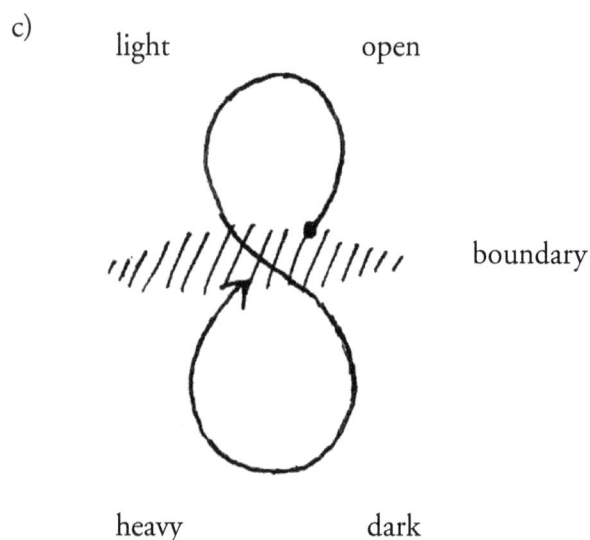

c)   light   open

boundary

heavy   dark

First in standing:
light zones – up - light
dark zones – down - heavy

then, with a 3/4 beat
then, with a 3/4 beat and
forwards/backwards;
thus, all 3 directions in space
up/down, right/left,
forwards/backwards

13. Harmonious Eight

Harmonious Eight

a) in standing
b) walking
c) turning around
   right/left
   Scales- Balance

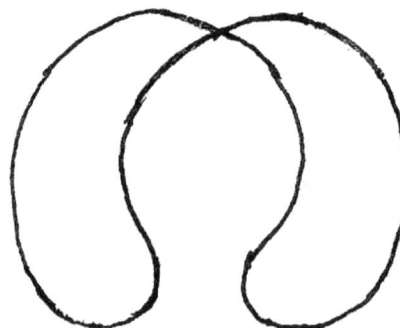

14. Harmonious Eight with 12 people *(even more directions in space)*

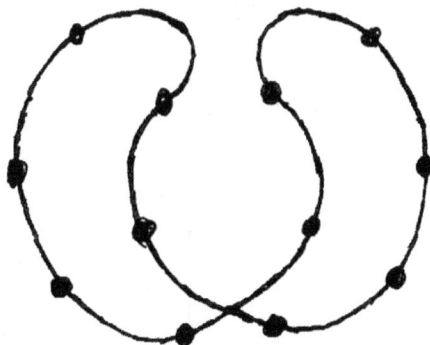

15. Variations of the Harmonious Eight *(Ilse Rolofs)*

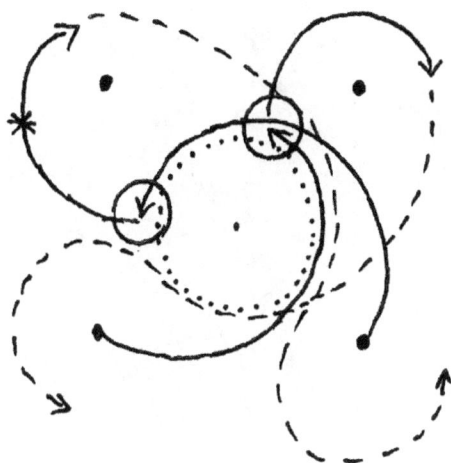

✳ : From here move backwards

◯ : At this point turn towards the center of the circle

16. Rod exercises for posture problems *(Ilse Rolofs)*

All rod exercises for posture problems in all three dimensions of space

1. Seven-part rod exercise: build up:

> a) in standing
> b) with the middle in-between
> c) with turning on the left
> d) the left is the middle, then the opposite.

2. Seven-part rod exercise: (generally good for thin "asparagus-like" children):

a) for the phlegmatic:

> down up
> down up   right
> down up   right left
> down up   right left   right
> down up   right left   right up
> down up   right left   right up   down

b) for the melancholic:

> down up
> down right
> down left
> down right
> down up
> down

c) for the sanguine (always the middle in-between)

> down middle – up middle
> right middle – left middle
> right middle – up middle
>   down

56

Three Versions

1) with a step in the middle and stand during the position
2) taking a step while going into the appropriate position (down, up...) and therefore standing in the middle
3) taking a step on performing both the position and the middle

a) for the choleric: The young choleric does it on a hexagon or six pointed star.

3. Rod Exercise

1) rod downwards (like in the 7-part rod exercise)
2) at shoulder height (stretched arms)
3) pulling in towards the chest (bent arms)
4) pulling out from the chest to shoulder height (stretched arms)
5) bringing downwards.

a) in standing
b) with 3-part walking (make sure that the feet and arms are well coordinated, moving together well)

4. Spiral Rod Exercises

With their variations along a spiral form, these are generally well known and good for general well being.

5. Throwing Exercises

a) throwing to a three-quarter beat, right – left – left, throwing between 3 & 1
b) pitch up/down, throwing on the change between up and down
c) rhythm (like throwing a spear) between back and forward

6. 12-part Rod Exercise

with 10 people

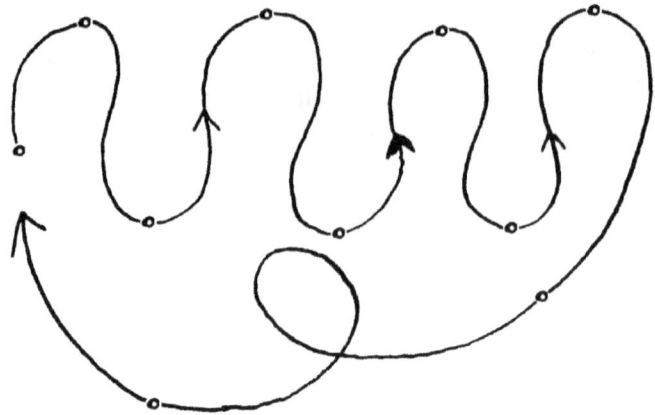

The streaming forces of the human being can generally be stimulated through these exercises and therefore by enlivening these forces, the spine can be strengthened indirectly and health-giving forces given to it.

General Foot Exercises

After extensive examinations of the feet, modern science (Professor W. Thomson) is convinced that due to negligence, or rather disfiguration of the feet, the organs of breathing and of circulation are affected. It is believed that due to atrophy (stunting) of the feet that have not been properly taken care of, a direct biological path can lead to a heart attack. Bent feet and other deformities of the feet happen mainly in childhood, generally without pain, and often can't even be corrected by orthopedic operations.

The threefold quality of the feet is mirrored in the threefold nature of the human body:

Firmness of the heels; sensitive toes; the balls of the feet to roll down with and the wonderful structure of the arches which allows the foot to be flexible and enter into weight as well as to free itself from it.

1. Big U exercise   Big I exercise

a) Feet in U: count to 12 while going slowly onto the toes then again count to 12 coming down slowly onto the heels

b) Rocking with the feet (from heel to toe)
   - 3 times forwards and backwards
   - 3 times adding an L that grows bigger and bigger using the arms
   - 3 times with the Growing L along an I or Ego-Line which increasingly gets longer
   - 3 times the Growing L on a circle which increasingly gets larger starting to the right (the circle should get smaller again as well)
   - 3 times the Growing L on a circle which increasingly gets larger starting over the left (the circle should also get smaller)

2. Doing the word "courage"

With children with feet problems you can also do the eurythmical gestures for the sounds in the word "COURAGE" because they tend not to be very courageous.

Exercises for Fallen Arches, for Splay or Spread Feet, and for Club Feet

(Ilse Rolofs)

1. N with the feet

a) in standing alternating between right and left.
b) while sitting using both feet at the same time.

2. M with the feet

a) In standing alternating between right and left.
b) While sitting alternating between right and left and then with both feet at the same time.

3. B with the feet

a) in standing alternating between right and left.

4. S with the feet

a) in standing alternating between right and left.

5. A with the feet, then U in standing

6. U

(Also for bed-wetting, hip problems, descended uterus, ticks and twitches and for people who get tired when standing)

U leads outwards with the help of buoyancy and an impetus to arise out of the heaviness. On the other hand incarnating creates a link to the earth through the legs and feet and brings the human being into himself.

7. U with rhythms

short – short – long
"So I do what is good
And with courage do too"

Either one steps the rhythm short–short-long, and then brings the feet together in a U, or else one pulls the feet together in a U already on the long syllable. After every short-short-long has been performed, bring the feet together in a U. For example: up onto the toes; from tip-toes downwards; or bending into the knees one or two jumps with the legs and feet together in U, etc.

(short-long-short) (short-long-short)
 Be   mer – ry   be   mer – ry

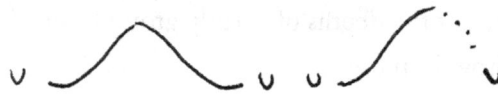

(short-long) (short-short-long)
 Go   up   in   the   air.

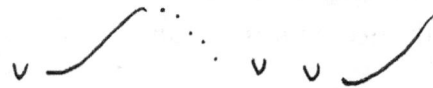

On the long, bring the feet together and go up on the toes with U. Go downwards on the following short. Take a step on the first short (as a concentration exercise alternate the starting foot between right and left.

8. C C C D

With children with fallen arches, with the D try to grow inwardly with a counter movement by going very slowly up onto the toes.

9. U in standing

We look	(feet together, arms upwards)
for the Good	(arms downwards)
We do it	(legs downward, bend the knees)
with courage	(upwards onto the toes)
We do it	(legs downward, bend the knees)
for fun	(U jumping up)
We do it well.	(legs downward; at the same time the arms in U upwards)
	(as a counter-movement: feet stretch upwards while the arms go downwards in U)

This is only one of many possibilities. After doing the exercise once through, it may be
done 6–10 times again with steps in order to enhance one's ability to concentrate.

To other texts:

Out of the depths of earthly ground
Grow I up towards heaven's round.

Out of the force of the root
Grows the tree towards the sun.

Fire flames in the blood
With strong courage you do!

Without rest or calm for you
Go to the goal, pursue, pursue.

The evergreen does upward grow
So calm and still the moon it shows.

(Text: Hedwig Diestel; see Appendices p. 197 for original German)

Exercises for Children with Splay or Spread Feet

1. Rocking

(To and fro 5 times,
then walking forwards only on the toes.
Rocking to and fro 5 times,
then walking backwards on the heels).

2. Three-fold walking

(On 1 lift roll the toes inwards, on 2 carry holding this contraction, carry the foot over the ground, and on 3 [place] stretch out the toes again into an I and place the foot).

3. Marble Game

(Grab a marble with your toes and toss it into a basket).

4. Walk

(On the outer sides of the feet (while experiencing a B).

Paralytics

With paralyzed patients Mrs. Rolofs always begins with N even if it's only in thought and imagination. N is the sound for destiny and since one cannot avoid one's destiny one must try to regain and re-enliven a connection to the earthly world.

a) I – with the feet: (right and left, first right,
   then left foot)

b) Light streams upwards,
   Weight draws downwards

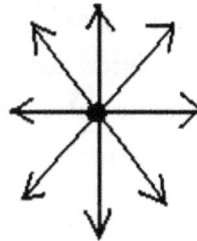

Exercises for a Child with Bow Legs
(Ilse Rolofs)

(Due to rickets there are deformities in the shoulders and the form of the head.)

1. I A O

2. Big Vowel Exercises A   U   I

3. Libra

zodiac gesture	consonant C	zodiac gesture
Gesture	Consonant	Gesture

4. L

at the end with the jump with X-legs, but in the beginning not with the jump

5. A

upwards T U like in Hope U

6. Courage

do the eurythmical gestures for the sounds in the word

7. Love-E

Let's observe cowards, people that are afraid. These are people who in their last lives weren't interested in anything. If we breeze through life superficially, not being interested in anything, then we can be sure that we'll be a scaredy-cat in our next life. This comes about when a disinterested or apathetic person doesn't unite enough with his surroundings then his future nerve-sense organism will have no sense of relationship to the earth forces. His bones remain undeveloped, his hair grows slowly and such people often have bow legs or knock knees.

—Rudolf Steiner, *Karmic Relationships,* Vol. II, Lecture 20

Exercises for Knock Knees or X-Legs

1. B

do many B gestures in standing and while walking

2. S

with O jump used against deformities in standing and walking

3. C-O-U-R-A-G-E

eurythmical gestures for the sounds

4. Love E

5. Big U

(classical big vowel exercise)

1. Writing with the feet (also for all other patients/cases)
2. Three-fold walking (normally, and with heaviness)
3. Running: (or having a race):

      a) on tip-toes
      b) on the heels
      c) alternating between toes and heels
      d) on the outer side of the feet

4. Copper balls or oranges between the feet or knees while walking
5. Picking up a small piece of veil or cloth with the toes
6. Toe-crawling exercise: forwards movement by doing a crawling movement with the toes.

Exercises to Achieve Agile Feet

In zig-zags:

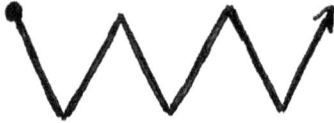

Diamonds

Silver-lights on tops of grasses
Sitting little pearls of dewdrops
How they glitter, how they shimmer
Glints of diamonds they are spraying.

These little grass blades
Enjoy their neighbors
Proudly shining
Those with tender sharp-like edges
Like in a king's crown glowing

(R. Hamerling. Translated from original German text, see Appendices p. 197)

Do it sideways beginning with the left foot. Over the right into the zig-zag and on the short syllables bring both feet together in U and go downwards onto the heels. When going in the right direction, the left foot begins. The other foot quickly joins the first in a U.

V. Children in Their Fourteenth Year

Around the age of fourteen the astral body lowers itself more and more into the physical body. The young adults at this age don't feel themselves to be quite at home in their own bodies. This is often due to the surrounding fat-layer which is missing from their physical bodies. They are often over-depressed and have overwhelming bursts of joy. Especially the girls at this age are always giggling. At this age minor thyroid-illnesses can arise. Girls often have an enlarged thyroid, which can lead to a real illness of the thyroid (loss of weight, the eyes protrude, the hands tremble, psychologically over-excited). The secretion of the thyroid gland allows for the development of the soul-life. It has a relationship to the etheric body. A person doesn't become an idiot because he can't think but because he is missing the instrument necessary for being attentive to his environment. A sympathy with and a true interest in things will be subdued if the thyroid is taken out. Other signs of disharmony and clumsiness can appear. Heart and/or breathing problems can occur at this time.

In any case one should try to help these young adults in their task of harmonizing the intervening, incarnating process of the astral body. The astral body must be in harmony and shine out because, according to Rudolf Steiner, the deepest causes of human illnesses lie within the astral body. (Many outer influences damage the astral body of these young people.) "As long as the person is unable to control his astral body himself, an angel being watches over it so that the uncontrolled forces do not completely destroy the astral body" (Rudolf Steiner). When the actual astral body is born at puberty, the cosmic-astral maternal sheath is released into the general astral world. The child must feel that the therapeutic eurythmist also knows something of this world. One talks to the child, explains the exercises to her. The child must feel that the therapeutic eurythmist understands her and that she can trust the therapist.

Thyroid Exercises

1. *"Light streams upwards..."*

2. *The pentagon*

3. *The hexagon*

4. *I A O*

5. *Harmonious Eight:* when done with 8 people

6. *Harmonious Eight:* with 12 people, but only in pairs (as in the form below)

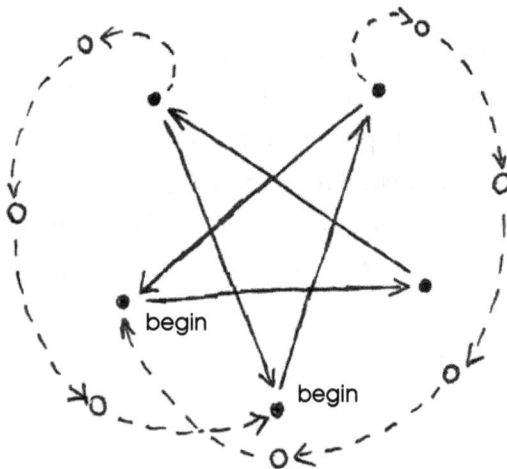

Inner way (pentagram)
I A O 3 x, then Outer way L

a) 3 times I A O on the pentagram (notice beginning places on previous page)
b) then five L's on the harmonious eight and five L's on the five pointed star.

7. _L M S_ (for thyroid problems) on a triangle

8. _S M I A_

earth triangle

heaven triangle

9. _Writing exercises_

"If one can't solve a problem, then one should try to change a letter in his/her own hand-writing." —Rudolf Steiner

10. Speech Formation exercises

(In doing these, pay special attention to the beginnings and endings of words and sharply distinguish them. If possible, practise these exercises several times a day.)

Leave no nickel
In what's given see inside!
Vulgar vagueness vary very vowing villain.
Better Betty and true to Trust.
Give bowing the gift to me.
Cold nickel lasting soon, and in clammy clothing.
Vain virtue visit silence; very vile will visit
He rescues riding the nicest rider reading the readiest rudder-retter.

(see Appendices p. 196 for this alliteration in German)

"The gentle pain that arises in the larynx by doing Speech Formation is diverted through our will to the body's periphery: the skin, the legs and the arms." —Rudolf Steiner

11. Kiebitz jump with M

12. Happy Eight with anapest

13. Evolutionary sequence

a) right arm
b) left arm
c) both arms
d) using objects

(alternating strengthens the etheric)

14. Alternating sequence Love-E and Light streams upwards

(Love-E, because most people with thyroid problems also have some kind of heart problem. Light streams upwards ... for children at least 14 years old so that the upper and the lower areas harmonize and grip into one another).

15. Mirror picture forms (*to strengthen morality*)

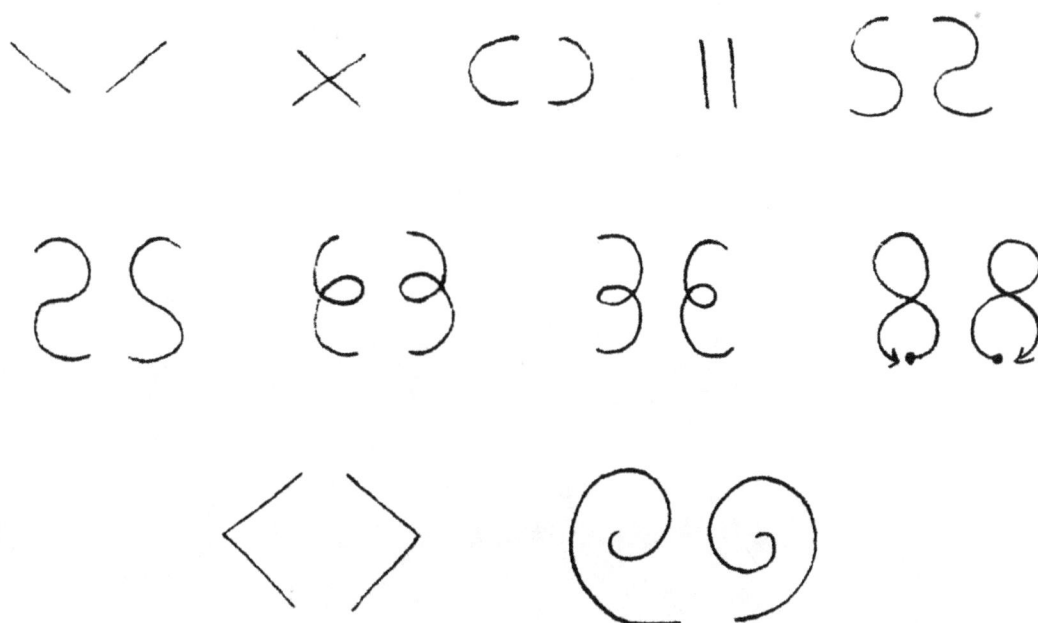

Do give special attention to the character and disposition of the person with a thyroid illness. Do those prepared exercises regularly and over a longer period of time: "Stay with it!" Try to dismiss such feelings as apathy, disinterest and lack of feeling.

From Conferences, January-September, 1924 in *Faculty Meetings with Rudolf Steiner: 1919-1924*, 2 vols. (Anthroposophic Press, Hudson, 1998) :

"The child does the therapeutic eurythmy exercises for a certain amount of time and these should be done daily."

"The child should be taken out of the classroom. If a child receives therapeutic eurythmy, then he is simply ill. Since therapeutic eurythmy is a therapy, the child may be taken out of any of the lessons except for the religion lesson. If he misses something then it's his karma. There can be no problems if one stands behind the importance of therapeutic eurythmy."

"There should be no teacher who does not appreciate therapeutic eurythmy so much so that he won't let the child leave his lesson."

"Unconscious repetition repeated over and over again, cultivates the feeling-life. Totally conscious repetition cultivates the actual true impulse of will since through that the power of decision becomes enhanced."

Disharmonious Conditions

VI. Hyperactive Children

Hyperactivity can be caused by minimal brain damage. In this case, call the child by his first name quite often during the lesson so that he comes into himself and doesn't lose himself in his surroundings. One therapist had good results from painting with the child before the therapeutic eurythmy lesson. Perhaps another child would need a different therapy before his therapeutic eurythmy lesson.

It can also be the result of an improper diet, for example from too much sugar (sweets) or food colorings or from preservatives.

1. Preliminary exercise: I A O

For harmonising the 3 parts of the organism; going from large to smaller movements has an incarnating effect.

a) With three-part walking:

   I arms upwards – A arms downwards – O arms middle

        lift   carry   place

b) One does I – A– O eurythmically but the intervals of the seventh,
   the third and the second are played musically
   (concordance) without the C as the prime.

c) I A O with the hands:
   Angel's I A O
   I with closed hands, palms facing one another like in U

d) I A O with the fingers

e) I A O while jumping with the feet

Do not use a text for the therapeutic eurythmy sequences of given sounds because the pictures conjured through a text only distract one from the true being of the sounds themselves.

2. Fidgety – iambus preliminary exercise

a) step an iambus thereby adding on more and more longs:

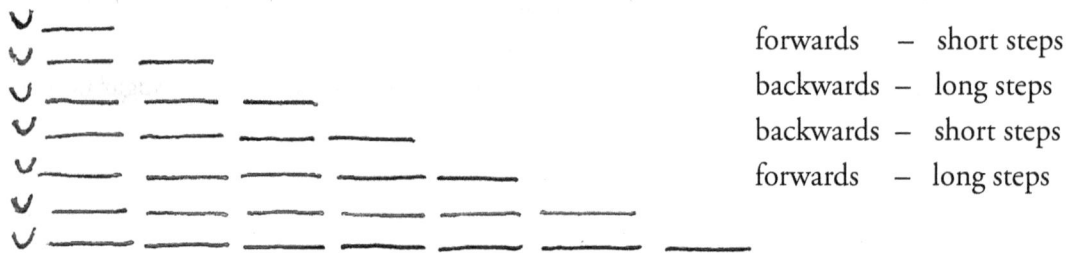

∨ ____	forwards – short steps
∨ ____ ____	backwards – long steps
∨ ____ ____ ____	backwards – short steps
∨ ____ ____ ____ ____	forwards – long steps
∨ ____ ____ ____ ____ ____	
∨ ____ ____ ____ ____ ____ ____	
∨ ____ ____ ____ ____ ____ ____ ____	

The important thing while doing this is to make sure that after the last long in each of the series, the foot which is behind is then placed next to that which performed the last long so that one may begin the next sequence with a proper short. The change of direction between short and long can be varied with as much fantasy as desired.

b.) Increase the shorts

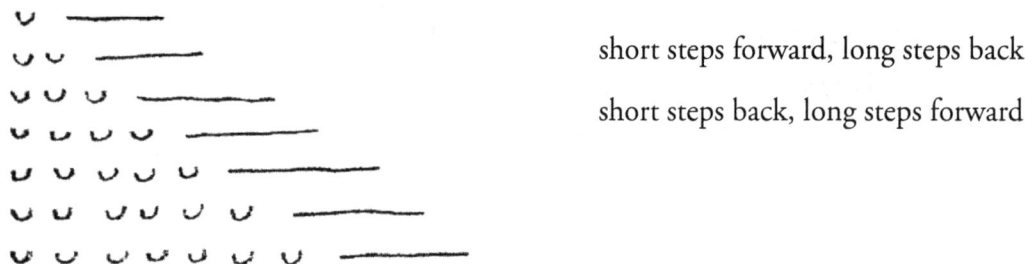

∨ ____	short steps forward, long steps back
∨ ∨ ____	short steps back, long steps forward
∨ ∨ ∨ ____	
∨ ∨ ∨ ∨ ____	
∨ ∨ ∨ ∨ ∨ ____	
∨ ∨ ∨ ∨ ∨ ∨ ____	
∨ ∨ ∨ ∨ ∨ ∨ ∨ ____	

Do this exercise continuously increasing longs or shorts up to seven times and then backwards again. In the beginning only do it three times. Add on more and more as the lessons go on.

3. Fidgety iambus *(as given by Rudolf Steiner)*

a) short – long: left – right, but do not emphasize either of the arms.
Mrs. Rolofs says, short – long and not left – right!
After the iambus let the arms go downwards to the sides of the body in Pause or Rest.

b) at first only the arms for a long period of time; sometimes with a different vowel such as E or U – practise for a long time. Then arms and feet together: that's already asking a lot! Do the arm movements very small at first so that the child doesn't excarnate any more than he already is.

c) I – move forward   (left arm forward and up, right arm, down and back)

   I – move backwards   (when moving backwards, take the sounds
   backwards too, down left behind, right up forward)

   O – Form sounds in the middle zone (backwards : O behind)

   U – Bring the arms together from outside towards the middle

d) Fidgety Iambus with Vowels:

for thin people who are fidgety	A
for people with back problems who are fidgety	I
for corpulent people who are fidgety	O
for people with problem feet who are fidgety	U

e) first towards the rod which the therapeutic eurythmist is holding

f) then without a rod

g) then from far apart, A going into a narrow U

77

4. Anapests on the circle and meander forms

a) On the circle, anapest to the left, then to the right

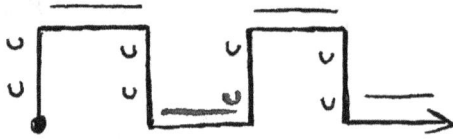

First the meander form
on the circle to the left,
then to the right. E
always on the long.

b) E middle, E above, E behind the back, and then E down (on the longs).
    (on form above)

5. Straight – curved: *(in forms)*

P

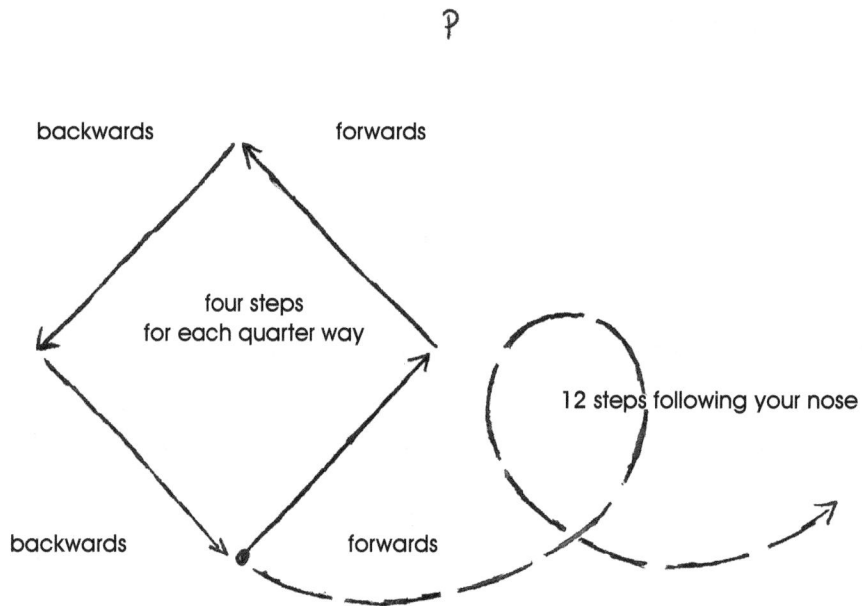

backwards   forwards

four steps
for each quarter way

12 steps following your nose

backwards   forwards

Square: At each corner after taking the fourth step bring the feet together and turn in the next direction. The first two ways following your nose; with the third and fourth way you are going backwards.

6. D F G K H *(the calming sequence given by Rudolf Steiner)*

a) in standing, very slowly

b) stepping

c)

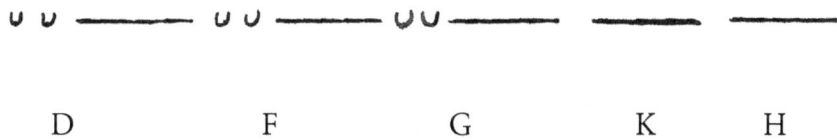

          D   F   G   K   H

Consonants on the longs

d) On an "I" or Ego- Line: D F forwards, G K H   backwards

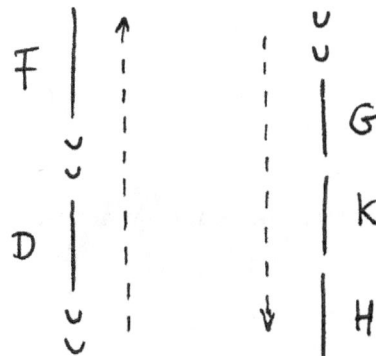

7. Stepping and maintaining balance

Turn the school desks over and use them as a balance beam. This is very good with such children.

8. *Transformation of the triangle*

First alone, then in pairs, then threes, each one starting from his/her place on the triangle.

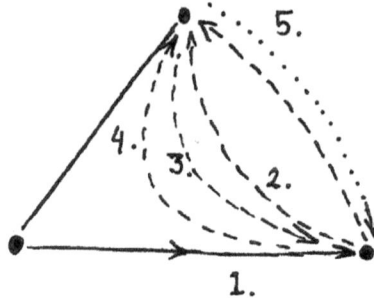

This exercise using triangles is good for concentration as well as for the social element, which is essential because these children need to work together to achieve social skills.

Take note the 5th way moves in the opposite direction: (very important for such restless children)

9. *Stepping an iambus to music*

With children always use the minor scale for iambic. When stepping a trochee, use a piece of music in a major key.

10. *Two forms of the "I" or Ego line*

a) Standing, do the Big E
     walking forwards, lead a large U towards the middle zone
     walking backwards, lead the U downwards

b) U walking forwards – middle zone
     N walking backwards
     B standing

11. If a child is in need of a particular soul attribute, such as courage or gentleness, etc., then it is suggested to have the child do the eurythmy gestures for the sounds for the word of that particular missing attribute in eurythmy a few times. Then, doing that word or words eurythmically without speaking it aloud at the end of the lesson.

12. Rod exercises

a) Lemniscate under the one knee and over the next, with steps.

b) Seven-part: always with a middle position in between:

Down	middle
Up	middle
Right	middle
Left	middle
Right	middle
Up	middle
Down	middle

c) Holding a rod horizontally in the hand, then toss it upwards and grab it with the same hand from above it. Then holding the rod horizontally with the hand and let it fall downwards thereby grabbing it from underneath.

d) Stretch arms over the head, then let the rod drop behind you and grab it from behind.

e) Finally, to the text:

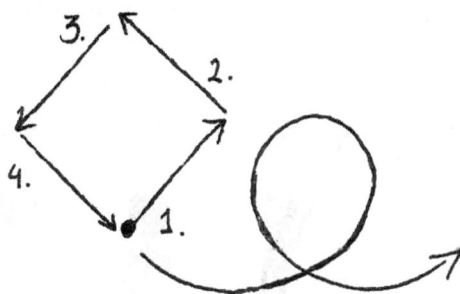

<table>
<tr><td>1</td><td>2</td><td>3</td><td>4</td></tr>
</table>

I go the way of courage and strength!

<table>
<tr><td>1</td><td>2</td><td>3</td><td>4</td></tr>
</table>

I want to find the Light in me

the loop form

That wins o'er Darkness victory!

With the rod: 1 right (like in the 7-part exercise)
2 up
3 left
4 down

All these exercises are to teach the child how to learn how to take hold of himself/herself and to give him/her some form.

The etheric body is stronger on the left side. The astral body is stronger on the right side. The rhythmical system becomes a-rhythmical when the nerve-sense system too strongly affects that which is surging upwards from the will-limb metabolic pole. That which is rising up from below breaks out and becomes independent and fidgety.

13. A upwards

U bring the lower arms (elbows) and hands together in front of the center of the body.

14. L U O K M (given by Rudolf Steiner)

3 times L; standing

U as in "I look upwards"; standing

O in the middle; walking backwards

K with a jump and the arms downwards; standing

M with both hands (the arms calming); walking forwards and then backwards

15. Coordination exercise

   I E I

a) alternating sides

b) arms and legs crossing:
    E with arms in front

c) arms and legs crossing:
    E with arms behind back

d) arms crossing E in front and legs behind.
    Then do the opposite:
    legs crossing; E behind the back

(the stretched arm or leg is always I)

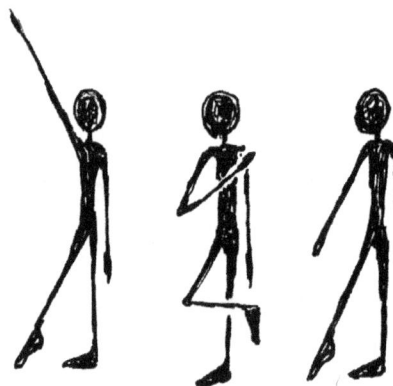

16. *D F G K H* + *R* (I Line - strengthens the sense of self)

a)

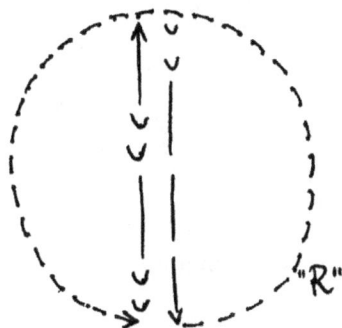 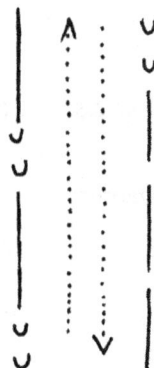

b)

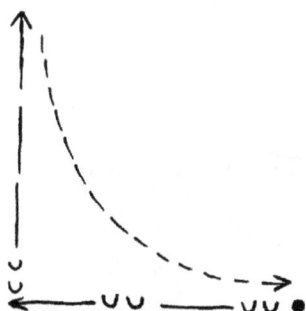

short-short-(D) long; short-short-(F) long (forward)   short-short-(G) long, (K) long, (H) long (backward)   R around in a circle

I-Line – strengthens the Ego

Use straight and curved lines to strengthen the etheric

c) This form for D F G K H in pairs (therapeutic eurythmist and child)

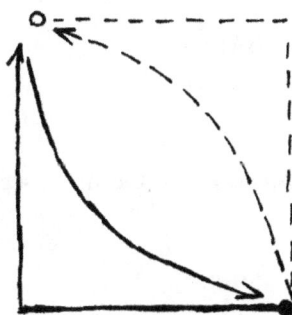

17. U for the hyperactive child

Bring the hands from way far out towards each other (the palms of the hands together, touching one another in U).

Big U Vowel Exercise: alter it according to appropriate age group

a) U hands together above the head leading downwards

b) U in the middle zone, from the sides bringing the arms together and downwards

c) U in the lower zone, from the sides bring the arms together and
   U go up on the toes and then down again

18. Exercises done backwards

Speaking the words of a short phrase or line of a poem

Poem on a five-pointed star, forwards and backwards: "The sun awakens worlds" done backwards would be: "Worlds awakens sun the"

1. The Sun awakens worlds
2. And sets the stars all dancing
3. To be part of the dancing whole
4. You too may join
5. Their dancing.

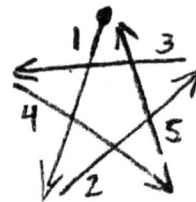

—A. Silesius (original German, see Appendices p. 197)

from The Bequest

1. I love the flame
2. The glow-element
3. In thunder and lightning
4. In stars-a-glimmer.

I love the ether,
The god-like freedom,
Where the winds, the clouds
And the eagles fly.

I love the waves
The splashing,
Longing, flowing,
From land to land.

I love the earth
That holy green
Where it's lovely to wander
And still sweeter to rest in.

Spirit shall flame,
Soul shall expand
The beating heart shall continue to sound and ring
The body shall rest.

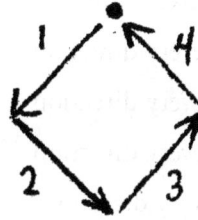

—R. Hamerling (original German, see Appendices p. 198

19. Exercises for directions in space

a) 5 steps in every direction
    4 steps in every direction
    3 steps in every direction
    2 steps in every direction
    1 step in every direction

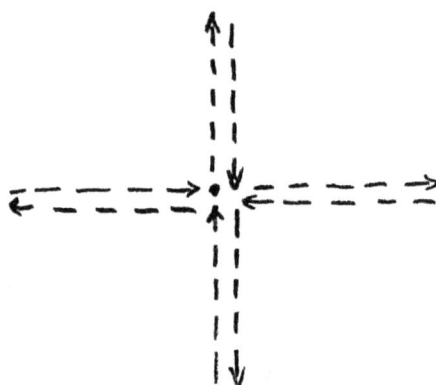

Also to :

Pease porridge hot,
Pease porridge cold
Pease porridge in the pot
Nine days old.

Some like it hot,
Some like it cold
Some like it in the pot
Nine days old .

VII. Chorea

Modern Pathology sees chorea as pathological disorder in movement, such as unmotivated muscle contractions that can only be suppressed for a short period of time, if at all and which hinder other movements. Unconsciously independent movements of the arms and legs appear. Especially characteristic of this illness are the contorted grimaces of the face and uncoordinated tongue movements which make speaking difficult. Despite these restless muscle contractions, chorea patients don't experience physical tiredness, although their psychological state is quite strongly affected. Their mental faculties are reduced and emotionally they easily become irritable. Colloquially, this illness is called St. Vitus's Dance and thereby suggestive of the past plagues of the Middle Ages, with which it has, however, nothing in common.

In fact this dance-frenzy of olden times, called St. Vitus, was a widespread epidemic disease that arose out of favorable breeding grounds of great physical and emotional suffering and which due to the character of the times gained the appropriate religious tinge. It went up in a fiery blaze and was generally over quite quickly. The evil began with an epileptic jerking of the entire body. Those who were affected lost consciousness and fell down. Then, their abdomen swelling and their mouth foaming, they would jump up and dance around. With uncanny distortions of their facial features, they would be seized for hours and hours in a wild fury, screaming and raging about until they broke down out of sheer exhaustion. They saw and heard nothing during this dance; immersed as they were in visions and in praising of the Divine. Their fit once over, they would moan and groan and complain until someone tied their abdomen tightly. Punches, kicks and pushes seemed to relieve them. Those affected by this illness behaved insanely and were looked upon as being possessed by evil demons such as those spoken of in the Bible.

This illness appeared for the first time between the eleventh or thirteenth centuries, and in the second half of the fourteenth century there was a tremendous epidemic. In July, 1374 the epidemic broke out in Aachen, Germany from where it spread to Cologne and then on to the Netherlands. In Cologne, it affected 500 people, in Metz, France 1100. It couldn't be stopped. Priests performed spiritual exercises trying to cure the sick. Those crazed with this "dance fever" were carried into the chapels of St. Vitus in Zabern and in Rothenstein so that they might be healed.

St. Vitus was martyred by the Roman Emperor Diocletian. The Feast of St. Vitus is celebrated on June 15. It is certain that St. Vitus has been mistaken for the slavic sun-god, Swantewit, whose temple in Ascona was converted into a chapel to St. Vitus by Christian monks in 879. When spoken, Swantewit sounds quite similar to St. Vitus. The festivities honouring Swantewit included dancing and fire, quite similar to our St. John's Festival, perhaps thus causing its mistaken affiliation to Saint Vitus's Dance.

Paracelsus was the first to deal with this illness. He put those with chorea in isolation, through which their suffering lost suggestive power. He also treated them with beatings and cold water. Later the complete opposite therapy was used. The dance frenzy was intensified in order to exhaust the patient as soon as possible. The town hired musicians to play so that those who were crazy about dancing (and such people were very receptive to music) would feel inspired to jump very high.

(from *The Dance* by Max von Böhn)

Around the age of 14, the astral body of the young adult must be able to enter into a well prepared physical body. This preparation begins at the age of seven. Those children with chorea are physically delicate and psychologically weak. These children distort their face with every emotion. Their in-breathing is also not in order. The whole physical organism is not being breathed through. Nothing reaches to the core. An imbalance exists between the etheric body and the astral body. The readiness to act is missing; the body is not permeable enough. Chorea can come about through shock, anger, and/or fear. The first symptoms of chorea are fluctuating changes of mood. The children don't feel well in their own bodies; they have slight breathing problems and start to stutter somewhat.

An important book in regard to this condition is *Das Geheimnis der menschliche Temperamente* [The Secret of the Human Temperaments] by Englert Fey.

Exercises

1. Bathing in I A O – in all variations

e.g.

Angels   I A O   (hands)
Butterfly I A O   (fingers)

2. Big A vowel exercise and Big U vowel exercise *(alternating 1 week long for each exercise)*

3. Jumping vowels   A E I O U   U O I E A

4. Five-Pointed Star with vowels *(to put the facial expression in order)*

– On every star-way a vowel: A E I O U
– After each star-way, M in standing:
– (thus A M A M I M O M U M)
  And thereby remain strongly in the feeling of the vowel A, E, etc .

5. Calming consonants

short – short – D   short – short – F   short–short – G, K, H with stamping
short – short-long   short-short-long   short-short-long-long-long

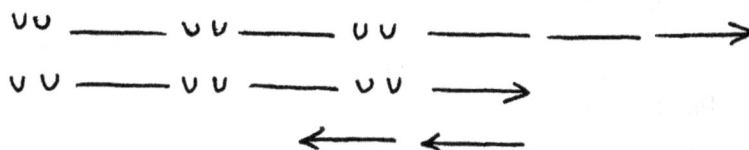

a) all going forwards

b) the same with stamping only on K H going backwards

c) On a five-pointed star (two people at the head and one at each other place)
All facing inward. One child at the head goes to the right foot with a D, the child at the right foot does a D at the same time, then he goes to the next place (left shoulder) with F. The child at that place (left shoulder) does F at the same time...etc.

d) D – F – G – K – H each on his own five-pointed star. On each corner one does the rhythmical R: D along the star-path, the rhythmical R in standing at the corner...etc.

6. *"He who shines through the clouds..."* *(on a five-pointed star)*

 May he illuminate, may he radiate, may he inspire
and fill with warmth and light, even us.

1. He who shines through the clouds:

    2. May   3. he illuminate

    4. May   5. he radiate

    6. May   6. he inspire

    8. May   9. he fill with warmth and light

                     10. even us

—Rudolf Steiner. (See Appendices p. 198 for complete German text of this verse.)

a. frontal

b. Pentagram ways, facing inward. "May" with a half-turn outwards; at the end, one looks again into the center.

This exercise is used "to develop the feeling and mood of honoring and admiring, and to acquire a sense of calmness."

(Rudolf Steiner to Tatiana Kisseleff)

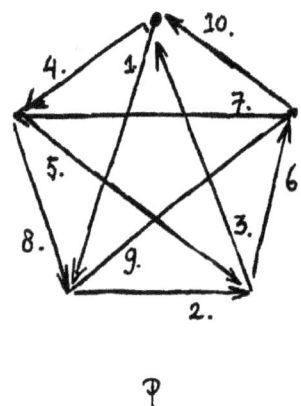

7. Happy Eight

Used "in order to develop a healthy feeling of joyfulness." (Rudolf Steiner)

8. Diaphragm O *(on the floor)*

– alternating with incarnating and excarnating spirals I A O U E

9. Verse of the Solstice *(on the hexagon)*

The Sun she turns around	(Sol revenit
The Earth is now joyous	Terre ridet
Through Darkness' blackness	Per tenebras
Espies she the light	Lux videt)

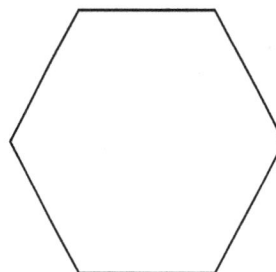

10. Forms with mirror images

Moving vowels on mirror form

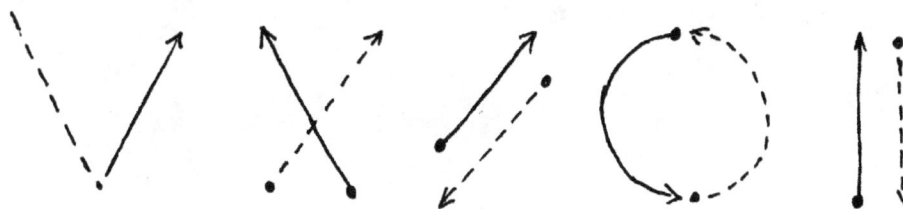

To enliven the will sphere: round forms

To enliven the thinking pole: straight forms

To enliven the feeling pole: round and straight forms

The therapeutic eurythmist begins, then the child does the mirrored image, then they repeat the forms simultaneously:

"The cross always wants to effect the transformation of the earthly into the spiritual. This will bring about the communion of the spiritual with the earthly." (Rudolf Steiner)

11. At the end of the lesson

– Reverence A (The children should feel themselves to be star children as in the Brothers Grimm fairy tale)

– T A O
– T I A O A I T

(do only the eurythmy gestures for the sounds without the form)

Concentration Exercises

1. Stepping forward and back

1 step forward	7,6,5,4,3,2,1 steps back
1,2 steps forward	6,5,4,3,2,1 steps back
1,2,3 steps forward	5,4,3,2,1 steps back
1,2,3,4 steps forward	4,3,2,1 steps back
1,2,3,4,5 steps forward	3,2,1 steps back
1,2,3,4,5,6 steps forward	2,1 steps back
1,2,3,4,5,6,7 steps forward	1 step back

a) On both the way forwards and backwards, begin on 1

b) On the way backwards, begin on 7
   (feet together after the last step in each sequence)

2. Variation

1 step forwards,	1 step backwards
2 steps forwards,	1 step backwards
3 steps forwards,	1 step backwards (until 7)

a) going backwards but doing the first step forwards

b) going backwards beginning with 7 steps and on 1 step forwards

3. Stepping while speaking (*"The child is good"*)

We can do all
We've fear of nothing,
We want to let
Our wings grow strong.

"One strengthens the child's will if the child speaks while walking without moving the arms at the same time." (Rudolf Steiner)

4. Alliteration

My beak is below
I burrow and nose
Under the ground,
I go as I'm guided...
(from an old English riddle: Plough)

5. Contrary rhythms *(the arms do the opposite of the legs)*

Rod Exercises

1. Place the rods in such a way as to form rays of the sun, towards the center.

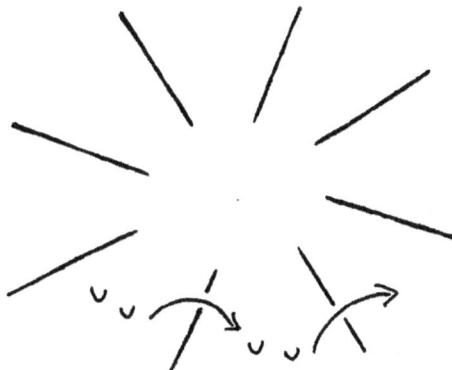

a) short – short - long   (do the "long" stepping over the rod)

b) long – short - short   (do the "long" stepping over the rod)

c) Place the rods closer together: short – long
$\qquad\qquad\qquad\qquad$ dwarf – giant

d) two children stand next to each other: one begins with the dwarf: the other with the giant.

e) the dwarves move counter-clockwise, the giants move clockwise along the circle.

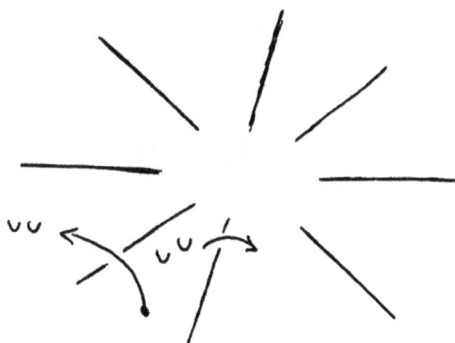

The dwarves make an E with their fingers and crouch down; the giants stretch themselves into a long I (this is an expansion /contraction at the same time).

2. Rod exercise *(with jumps)*

Seven-part rod exercise:

With feet together jump in the directions of the arrows: down - jump forwards;
up – jump backwards; right – jump to the right, etc.

3. Rod exercise *(in 3/4 beat)*

1. the rod to the right: while taking a step with the foot to the right
2. toss the rod over the head and catch it with the left hand: while taking a step with the left foot to the left
3. lead the rod vertically towards the middle: bring the left foot to meet the right.

4. At the end of the lesson

- TAO
- TIAOAIT (only the sounds, not on the form)

VIII. Rocking or Swaying To and Fro

Usually these are very intelligent and gifted children with delicate nerves. They might rock from right to left or forwards-backwards. People with this rocking phenomenon remain as if in the sphere of the moon, not wanting to incarnate. One child, 6 years old, rocked himself from the right to the left and hummed to himself. This began about midnight and increased in intensity until the morning. During the day he was very pale.

1. *I I S S R R*

Before the exercise: I – stretching (left – right)

                            S – (left – right) from up to down with anapest

                            R – continuously, from down to up, without rhythm

a) I left   –   with a step to the left

    I right   –   with a step to the right

    S left   –   with a step to the left (from above downwards)

    S right   –   with a step to the right

    R left   –   left forward, with a step to the left; to the side

    R right   –   right forward, with a step to the right; to the side

b) Original exercise for rocking and swaying (from Rudolf Steiner)

left arm	I	right arm	I
left arm	S	right arm	S
left arm	R	right arm	R

Do this for a long time until the child really sweats. Dr. Kirchner: These children are very much connected to their mothers. The therapeutic eurythmist Mrs. Wallerstein had the patient do this exercise for 10 minutes. She did the "U" from wide apart and then together and she did concentration exercises as well.

c) then this same exercise as above in a) only jumping with the feet and to the sides instead of taking a step.

2. The whole Big A vowel exercise

3. Five-pointed star getting smaller

1. all star ways with 5 steps along each way, then 1 step into the middle
2. all star ways with 4 steps along each way, then 1 step into the middle
3. all star ways with 3 steps along each way, then 1 step into the middle
4. all star ways with 2 steps along each way, then 1 step into the middle
5. all star ways with 1 step along each way.

Then taking one step into the middle and there standing still while inwardly letting the exercise echo into your entire being:

4. *A A U* (*A down in the arms, while moving forwards in the space*)

A upwards with the arms while going backwards in the space

U beginning in the middle sphere going downwards with the arms together, then in standing tap your hands against the soles of the feet (right hand against the left foot, left hand against the right foot)

5. *T U B A*

T – on the head
U – with the backs of the hands together lead the arms downwards
B – around the middle of the torso
A – with the arms all the way down

a) all the consonants and A with the arms and the legs

b) all the consonants and A with the arms going downwards while jumping with the legs.

6. Contraction and expansion

"Annoy me not, leave me in peace   (Stand on the contraction, then
I have not strength nor courage least   run back and expand, then
I'll laugh at you and I go home   contract again in the
to rest within myself alone."   finishing position)

(See Appendices p. 198 for original German version.)

Do this exercise as if standing over and above everything.

Two children stand across from one another; stamping 4 steps forwards while doing a contraction with their torso and arms. During the next 4 longs (the 2nd line) do an A with the arms, expanding. Turn and go outwards with the 3rd line. Turn and in standing do a contraction to the 4th line.

7. T I A O A I T

T   above

I   stretching upwards first to the left then to the right
    (with the transition to the right)

A   all the way to the back and sensing the moment of passing through the I position in
    the vertical and into the O forwards

A   again behind as described above

I   upwards to the right   also in reverse order

I   upwards to the left

T   above

8. Harmonious Eight rod exercise

a) Holding the rod in the right hand, the left hand does the mirror image:

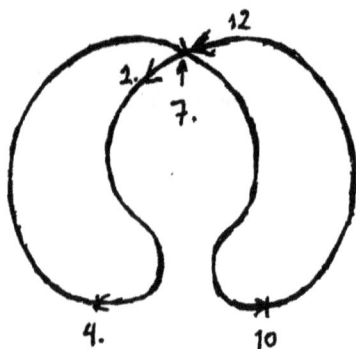

On 4 and on 10 do a half turn on the circle as in the drawing. We go along the large circle in the room. On 7 change the rod into the other hand over your head. For the whole exercise count to 12 beginning above and to the right.

With very difficult cases of rocking and swaying

Lightly massage the right and left side of the child's backbone with salt from the Adriatic Sea, preferably when the salt contains some specks of gold. (Indication from Rudolf Steiner)

9. Rod exercises

Loop (an open eight) – a connection to the cosmos

(from above)

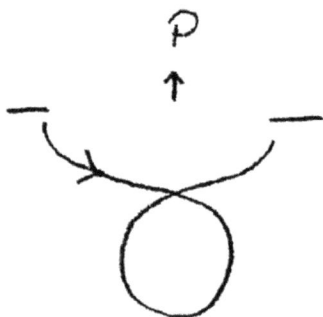

begin above to the left, then towards oneself and end above to the right.

IX. Children Damaged Due to Environmental Conditions

Exercises for Frail Children

(who generally feel dizzy, nauseous and/or tired)

Ilse Rolofs "bathed" these children in five-pointed star exercises.

1. I A O

2. Classical big E-exercise

3. Pentagram with I A O

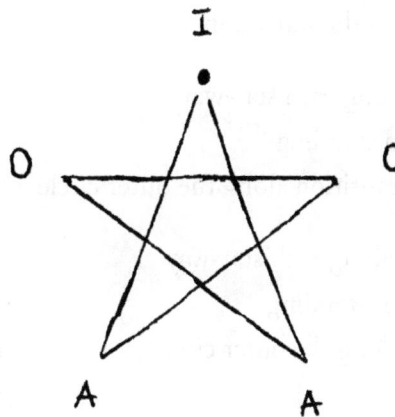

Changing directions strengthens the etheric body.

4. *Five-pointed star* (frontal)

a) L along each star-way
    M in standing   (to bring warmth into the child)

b) I along each star-way
    L in standing   (to bring steadfastness)

c) A along each star-way
    B in standing   (to give courage)

5. *Five-pointed star* (all looking towards the center)

a) L along each star-way   M in standing
    B on the transition (along the outer dotted circle)

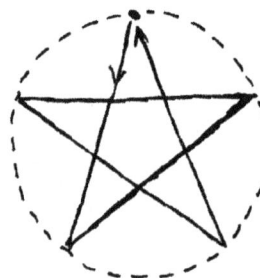

b) I along each star-way
    L in standing
    B on the transition

c) E along each star-way
    B in standing
    I transition along the outer circle

d) L along each star-way
    M in standing
    O along the outer circle   (with children who are easily exhausted,
                                              do L M O; this pushes the etheric body
                                              together into a oneness)

6. *Five-pointed star* (but as a Crown Form with 5 children)

L along each star-way, but continuously
growing from small to large

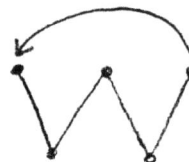

7. Anapest *(also as a mirror-image)*

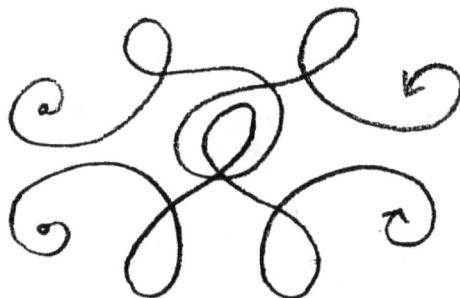

8. Four leaf clover form

a) one stands in a square:
   (to strengthen the heart)

b) E G along the lemniscate
   L and M as the transition

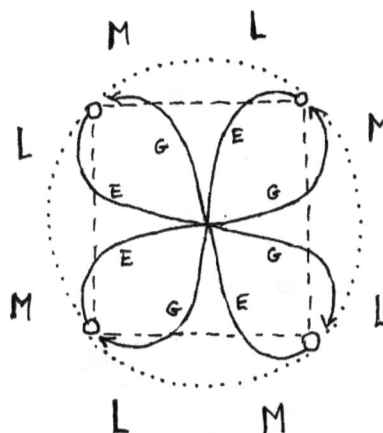

9. Lemniscate *(in different directions)*

3 steps along every 1/4 of the lemniscate
(=12 steps for each completed lemniscate)

a) always frontally

b) following your nose

c) always with your back towards the
   middle of the form:

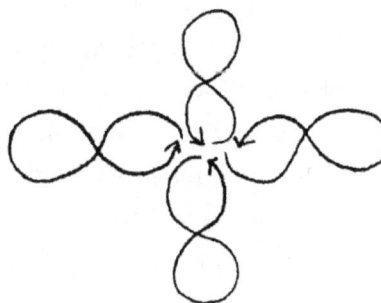

Exercises for Children with Vitamin D Deficiencies

From a lecture by Rudolf Steiner of March 14, 1909 in Hamburg: "Der Kreislauf des Menschen innerhalb der Sinnen-, Seelen- und Geisteswelt" (Human Circulation within the Worlds of the Senses, the Soul and the Spirit):

"Look at the child: After a child is born, he has developed certain parts of the brain which one can call sense-centers or nerve-networks. These are already developed within the first week of life. On the other hand, if you were to examine the brain at the end of the first month, then one would see that almost two thirds of the brain had developed only within the previous four weeks. Little by little the inner two thirds of the cerebral cortex fills up with nerve substance which allows for the connection between one sensory impression and the other. The child sees colors and hears tones but cannot yet connect them. The nerve strands which convey these sensory impressions are being developed little by little."

"Inflammation of the heart can occur often in adolescence as a result of overdosing with vitamin D)."—From Dr. zur Linden, *Erfahrungs-Heilkunde*, Volume XVI, Feb. 1967, Vol. 2 .

Is damage due to vitamin D overdosing curable?

Professor A. Beuren first warned of the dangers of vitamin D damage at a congress for Pediatricians (May 6-8, 1966). He said that vitamin D is not a remedy but only a substitute substance. Rickets is a disturbance of the metabolism of light due to the sick child's inability to complete the transformation of the pro-vitamin D into the end product vitamin D either because he hasn't enough sunlight or because he lacks the capacity to complete the metabolic process. This pro-vitamin is found in subcutaneous fatty tissue as long as this is not removed by daily bathing or showering with soap (which is harmful). Excessive vitamin D causes an abnormal acceleration of the mineralization processes in the child's skeletal and vascular systems.

Normally the physical body of a newly born child contains about 12% less mineral salts than of an adult. This small leeway will slowly diminish over the years, which is a part of the natural aging process. In the course of this gradual and continuous deposition of mineral salts, the child proceeds naturally through the stages of his development in to adulthood. The life rhythms in which the child learns to grip, to stand upright, to crawl, to stand, to speak and finally to think are directly related to this progression. Into this regular process, the effects of vitamin D doses force their way in to the child in a most dubious manner. The above-mentioned life rhythms accelerate and thus the biological aging process progresses too swiftly. Premature acceleration of later stages of development can lead to an insufficient development of the organs, causing functional weaknesses in later years.

About Children with Problems Caused by Excess Vitamin D:

(some observations from over four decades)

Children not affected by excess vitamin D: blooming with vitality, less nervousness, more resistance against infections, and a joyful sensitivity. They have a better bone structure with less matter in the tissues and are less heavy.

Bad eating habits have just as bad an effect; for example condensed milk, powdered milk preparation, and in general, convenience food products for children.

Children affected by excess vitamin D mature at an early age and are precocious at the expense of forces which are otherwise reserved for the future. This as well as an inharmonious maturing of the integration of body and soul is fostered by the overdose of vitamin D.

"Our treatment for rickets, if need be already in a child's first 5–6 weeks of life, using Phosphorus as well as Calcium I and II (Apatitee 6x Comp. and Conchae 5% Comp.)"

Excess vtamin D leads to the calcification of the blood vessels of the heart, the kidneys or of the brain, and as a further extension of these circulatory problems the child in his habits comes to resemble an early maturing adult. In a clearly negative way a change appears in consciousness, at present usually only after 9 or 10 years old: diminished performance at school, lack of interest, poor concentration, decreasing desire to learn, and a restriction of spiritual horizons to purely technical areas, all in contrast to those children who are not affected by excess Vitamin D. It is also not desirable for pregnant mothers to take excess vitamin D. Of course, excess vitamin D alone is not always responsible for these conditions, but one can more easily recognize and deal with it than the other possible factors.

For problems due to excess vitamin D, one can take some additional medicine, such as plumbum met. (metallicum) 4%

Degenerative kidney disorders, heart defects, inflammation of the heart or diabetes with children of otherwise healthy families could be the result of excess vitamin D. The extent of the damage caused by it can go from hardening of the vessels and calcification of the bones to advanced anatomical changes in the aorta or of the vessels of other organs such as the kidneys, the pancreas, and the brain. The consequences can lead to inflexibility in one's thinking, to poor concentration, to retarded intellectual development, to strong mineral deposits within the child's tissues, and/or to a coarseness of the skeletal system. Heart attacks among youth could also belong in this area. At the time of this conference in 1971, the U.S.A., Russia, and other countries had not addressed vitamin D-related illnesses.

The teachers only complained about "a shocking deterioration in children's performance at school."

Exercises

1. L *with increasing steps*

L 1,   L 1 2,   L 1 2 3,   L 1 2 3 4   etc.

Their performance at school is worst at the ages of 10, 11, or 12.

2. Pentagram exercise *(He who shines through the clouds)*

(Variation of earlier exercise on p. 90)

1. He who shines through the clouds	on each star way:
2. May he	3. illuminate
4. May he	5. irradiate
6. May he	7. inspire
8. May he	9. fill with warmth
	10. us also

a) frontally

b) do star-ways while facing the center of the star. Do "May he" turning with a semi-circle to face outwards and at the end return facing towards the middle again.

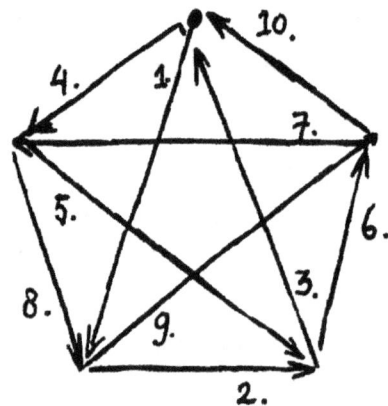

106

3. In cases of dizziness / problems of balance

A lemniscate lying horizontally, beginning slowly and then getting faster until it becomes a quick walk. At the end strongly clap the hands together and clap against the soles of the feet as well:

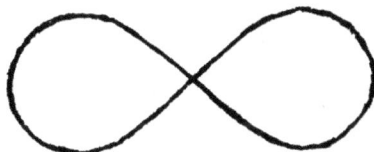

4. An exercise for the rhythm of the heart

(short – short – short – short – long)

Do only with children who are at least 9 years old.

Do the 4 shorts as 4 steady, small steps while measuring (taktieren) the width of the torso (from shoulder to shoulder) with the arms. On the long do one long smooth step especially using the foot while leading the arms quietly downwards and then gently upwards again to the height of the shoulders (the down-up under one long).

Exercises for Sleeping Disorders

1. Incarnation and excarnation spirals *(for both, the sounds A O U E)*

This exercise was given by Rudolf Steiner.

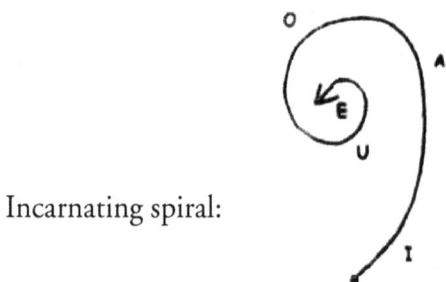

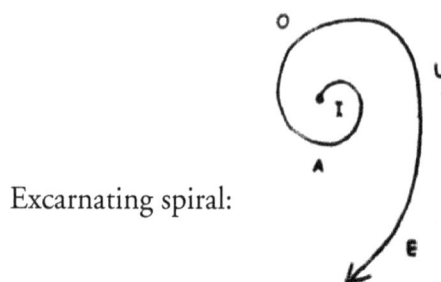

Incarnating spiral:

Excarnating spiral:

I coming from heaven	I inwards into oneself
A coming more and more	A getting continuously larger
O into oneself	O
U like a T on the chest (feeling a U between the backs of the hands)	U arms upwards with palms of hands together
E being completely within oneself	E with outstretched arms like Christ on the Cross, breathing out

2. Solstice verse *(Sonnenwendspruch)*

1. The Sun she turns about	(Sol revenit
2. The Earth is rejoicing	Terre ridet
3. Through shrouded darkness	Per tenebras
4. Discovers the light.	Lux videt)

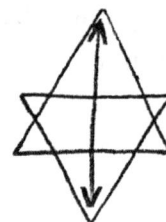

Alternative translation of poem from p. 89.

a) (this is to be done just before and just after the Solstice Verse)

3 times L - paths along the heavenly triangle
1 time A - a straight line forwards
3 times L - paths along the earth triangle
1 time I - a straight line backwards

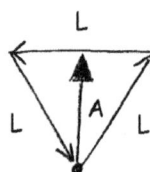

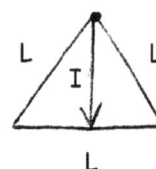

108

Exercises for Bed-wetters

"Within such children who are bed-wetters lies a wounded soul."
(from R. Steiner, *Education for Special Needs,* Rudolf Steiner Press, London, 1998)

The therapeutic eurythmist must try to acquire the child's trust. One must look into the possibility that the child might be yearning for a dear relative who has died.

Ilse Rolofs spoke with a child about what happened to him in the night. She asked the child to tell her when urination happened by nodding or shaking his head, so that it wouldn't be so embarrassing for the child.

She asked the mother to make up the bed afresh for the child and to give him clean sleepwear so that the child in his unconsciousness wouldn't want to dirty the clean bed sheets. If the sheets and/or clothes smell at all of urine, then the child unconsciously feels himself to have returned to his former state of babyhood.

1. *"An hysterical flying out" of the astral body*

a) allow them to run, then stop abruptly

b) let them hop or skip, then with the sounding of a gong they must stop abruptly

2. *Contraction and expansion*

Contract backwards, expand forwards (Ilse Rolofs)

a) first do large movements, then let them become smaller

b) then only do the movements with the hands

c) then do the movements with each single finger

3. L B U – L B I – L B N

a) L forwards
    B back
    U standing

b) L forwards
    B back
    I standing

c) L forwards
    B back
    N standing

d) U forwards
    B back
    N standing

e) E (big) standing
    U forwards
    U back (downwards)

4. "He who shines through the clouds" on a five-pointed star

(cf. Exercises for children with problems caused by excess vitamin D)

—Rudolf Steiner (See Appendices p. 198 for complete German Text of this poem.)

5. The expanding vowel circle A, E, I, O, U

(This is similar to the picture of the bladder contracting and becoming slack.)

6. Classical A exercise (Venus and the sound related to the kidney)

7. Love-E

because often these children have been deprived of something or someone that they otherwise would have had.

8. F-exercises

Ilse Rolofs has had good experience with using B and A when such children do not react well to the F.

a) F with a jump (but be very strict and make sure that the child brings it back towards himself.) If you are working in a Children's Home, then practise B in the morning and F in the evening with them.

b) "Bed-wetter F": (from an older eurythmist who had worked in a school) For the first part of the F slap the hands on the thighs, then bring the F downwards and forwards. Then bring the hands back and pull in the fingers. Do the same movement while jumping on the toes. Then bring the arms back towards you with the fingers bent inwards and go slowly down onto the heels of the feet.

c) One can jump forwards with many strong Fs one after another without a pause in between and then go down very slowly from the toes onto the heels. After this a good long pause.   By performing the F, one must activate the out-flowing because these children hold back their urine during the day and let it go at night. One must take hold of the warmth-organism within the F. In the fire-process, form is retained within the element of warmth.

d) F: practise first the thrusting, then form a curve like in the gesture for R but remain contained within oneself and do not lean outwards or forwards into the movement but rather like covering over something.

e) F downwards:

But as if the whole body were shaking. Then breathe out a warmth downwards while bringing the palms of the hands towards the body. The hands should be rounded as if forming a covering. One should let the warmth stream through the whole child; even into the thighs, knees, calves, and feet.

With the F-Jump on the toes: jump so lightly that the F could fly and spray out of the heels of the feet from behind, then slowly and warmly place the heels onto the floor. Emphasize and cultivate this sense for the warm inner space in the arch of the feet.

The F is a reaction to a stormy environment. Rudolf Steiner performed F downwards but very elastically because he brought it softly upwards again. (Do this shaking as if shivering throughout the body. Then, instead of going upwards elastically with the arms, breathe out and downwards while bringing the arms towards the body but do not pull them back towards the body stiff and cramped.)

"Here we have the sound F. This has to do with something 'psychic'. One must try to perform the jump in such a way: one begins to make the jump and tries to go forwards but now at the moment of landing one comes down quite strongly onto the toes, then brings the heels down, once again jumping on tip-toes and then coming down onto the heels. It would be exactly the same in the case of the (German) V (which is pronounced like a soft F in English). Here we have a movement which should be practised when one finds that the process of urination is not in order. It is naturally always possible to combine the movements in the most various ways for one will find in the doing of them that one needs to do the one or the other in combination in one or the other direction."

(Rudolf Steiner, Curative Eurythmy Course, lecture 4.
Rudolf Steiner Press, London, 1983)

f) F with a copper rod: Hold the rod horizontally; go with an F gesture downwards to the thighs pulling the rod in close to the body (such children are very unconscious in this area).

9. Reverse order exercise *(Rückshau)*

1, 121, 123, 121, 1234, 123, 121, etc.

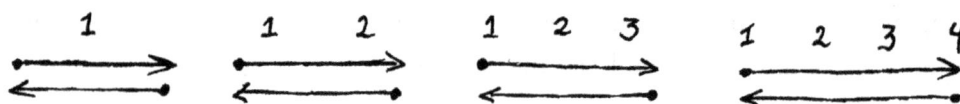

10. Footstool exercise

Standing on top of a footstool: jump down, landing on the toes and then slowly going down onto the heels. Then with the legs very tight together, jump forwards five times and then backwards five times. The ankles and feet should be well pressed together.

11. The B–A–B–U–B

a) B with the arms, well-enclosing B with the legs; they should not extend over the middle of the body: (the body's symmetry-line)

b) A with the legs, then going up onto the toes but taking care that the shoulders remain quiet and at the same height, at the same time bend the knees without going onto the heels. One remains at one's normal height.

c) B then place a small stone on the floor and with a gesture of protection enclose the stone with your foot. The arch of the foot builds a house around the stone. (One must create an inner space for bed-wetters.)

d) U bending into the knees (such children are terribly stiff from their hips downwards) Bed-wetters are often children who are poorly incarnated in their feet and often unconscious of their body from the hips down. In this case it is advisable to do feet massages, eurythmy exercises with the feet and U bending into the knees.

e) B from above the head going downwards bending into the knees. When possible, practise with B in the morning and F in the evening.

12. Forwards – Backwards movement: LBU LBI LBN

a) L forwards
B backwards 3x
U standing on the toes

b) L forwards
B backwards 3x
I standing on the toes

c) L forwards
B backwards 3x
N with a jump back

13. Big classical A-exercise

14. B T U (Hysteria Sequence)

15. Evolutionary Sequence

B M D N R L, etc., with copper balls in the hand, so that the movement does not flow out.

Exercises Relating to Undescended Testicles

1. A – U *(A upwards — U pulling in together in the forearm)*

2. U – A *(U upwards, then A leading downwards until A with bent knees; Jumping with A many times consistently holding this position in the legs)*

Little Froggie hop, hop, hop
Little Froggie stop, stop, stop

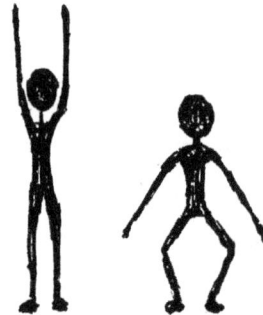

3. "Big Boy" exercise

a) Take an A upwards and, while standing and leaning against a wall, a U downwards towards the outstretched legs which are in A.

b) Child sits with his back pressed
against the wall and does A with
the legs outstretched on the floor,
A bringing the arms up over the head,
U with the arms and the head leading
downwards towards the floor
into the already stretched out A-legs.

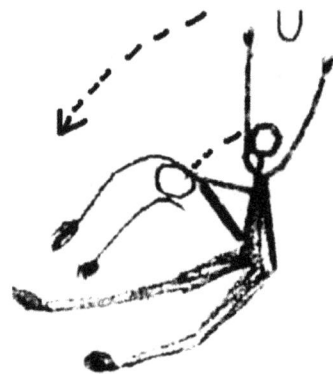

4. Standing in U *(bend into the knees taking the arms downwards in U)*

5. Standing in I *(stretching the leg out to the side and then bend the knee of the standing leg)*

Alternate between right and left if both testicles are raised; otherwise do only that side where the testicle hasn't dropped.

6. D and T *(with jumps going down lower and lower)*

7. Alliteration practice with the legs

8. K *(with a jump)*

9. G K D T R *(jumping with each consonant – Dr. Carl Nunhofer)*

X. Stuttering

Speech impediments and stuttering occur when one cannot carry out during this earthly life those intentions which one had decided upon while in the spiritual world before birth.

Dr. Karl König: "Stuttering is a kind of epilepsy of the larynx. The in-breath is cramped and the out-breath is jammed or congested. In the case of epilepsy the astral body is cramped within the human organism."

Exercises (Ilse Rolofs)

As children in Waldorf Schools would often speak verses and say prayers, Ilse Rolofs preferred to work with the pure sounds rather than use verses.

1. Hexameter

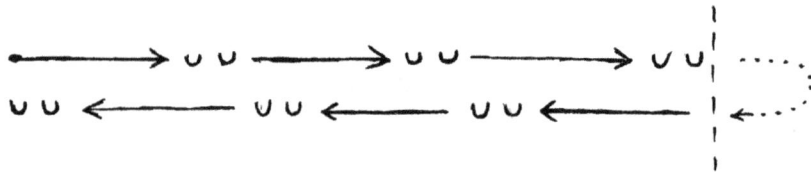

long – short – short – long – short – short – long – short – short /
long – short – short – long – short – short – long – short – short

a) Three dactyls going backwards with the sound which is stuttered (G K A I), then in the caesura a one-syllable word with the stuttering-sound and three dactyls going forwards.

b) Then three dactyls going backwards with A E I (in-breathing) then three dactyls going forwards with I O U (out-breathing). Do this on a lemniscate form (in the caesura, one doesn't move; this is like a streaming into the soul, into the body and then streaming into the world; the caesura is oriented accordingly.

c) Then while going backwards on three dactyls L L M and while going forwards on three dactyls: M L L

d) Then while going backwards on three dactyls: A A I (in-breathing) and while going forwards on three dactyls: I O O (out-breathing)

2. Vowels *(practice them the way they are naturally formed in the mouth)*

A E I O U   U O I E A

forwards   backwards

a) speaking

b) then with the arm gestures (forwards and back)

c) then with the arm gestures while moving forwards and backwards

d) then with the arm gestures while jumping forwards and backwards

3. Speaking exercise K L S F M

(From Dr. Rennefeld, who may well have received this exercise from Rudolf Steiner.)

a) speak all the sounds loudly on one full out-breath, so that by M the breath is used up

b) speak quietly

c) whispering

d) only in thought

e) then, once again let the sound resound (in a normal voice)

f) then do the exercise loudly with all the vowels. A E I O U

Dr. Rennefeld: "Stuttering is fear that has entered the physical organization. Therefore one must strengthen the out-breathing: K L S F M on one entire out-breath."

4. On an in-spiralling form I A O U E *(U pointing towards the heart)*

5. On an out-spiralling form I A O U E *(U upwards; ending with the big E like a cross)*

6. Rocking L *(forwards-back-forwards while stepping forwards; backwards-forward-backwards while stepping backwards)*

Do this while doing a large but normal L.

7. E – L E – L

Along the figure of a lemniscate as indicated, finishing with G on the circle and always while looking towards the center of the circle.

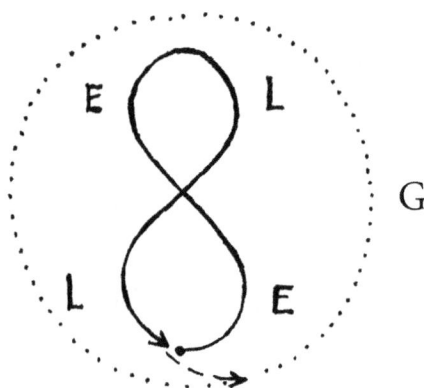

For a boy who first began to speak at the age of three or four and who only after the age of five could first barely speak full sentences with a tendency to stutter, shake his head and wet the bed (an insufficient formation of the head-chest region), Rudolf Steiner gave the following exercises: G K A I as well as exercises with dumb-bells in order to enhance the sense of balance.

In the therapeutic eurythmy course (Stuttgart, June 14, 1920) Rudolf Steiner said that nervous children who stutter had to practise with K and P. They had to speak, walk and do sentences in eurythmy with K and P.

"Stutterers don't have enough self-leadership nor are they in command of their incarnation."

Rudolf Steiner on stuttering

The Child's Changing Consciousness as a Basis of Pedagogical Practice, Lecture 2 (Anthroposophic Press, Hudson, NY, 1996)

Speech and Drama Course, CW 282 (Anthroposophic Press, Hudson, 1986). Steiner speaks about the labial and dental consonants and goes on to speak about lisping and stuttering.

The Renewal of Education, CW 301, Lecture 12 (Anthroposophic Press, Hudson, NY, 2001). Steiner speaks about breathing and its connection to stuttering.

Curative Eurythmy, (Rudolf Steiner Press, London, 1983)

Further Exercises

1. Frau Baumann, therapeutic eurythmist

a) contraction and expansion

b) yes and no exercise

c) hexameter

d) veneration-A

e) out-winding spiral

2. Dr. Ott

a) 3 x L horizontally while walking backwards
    M once, using both hands in a forwards direction but while walking backwards

b) The therapeutic eurythmist and the child hold one another's hands like in Ree-ra-ragon, we're riding in the wagon; in the wagon we are riding: ree rah ragon: (standing side by side, both cross their arms at the wrists and take hold of the other's hands therefore the right hand holds the partner's left hand and the left hand holds the partner's right hand.)

3. Isabelle De Jaager, therapeutic eurythmist

a) D F G K H on an in-winding spiral form

   L M N P Q on an out-winding spiral form

   For sanguine children, do both sequences while stepping short - short – long

   For phlegmatic children, do both sequences while stepping long – short – short.

b) To a Hexameter I O A, then the caesura,

   – and after the caesura, reverse A O I

   – do the same using L M S - caesura - S M L

One should let the child do the eurythmic gestures of those consonants that he cannot speak.

4. Frau Kugelmann and originally from Rudolf Steiner

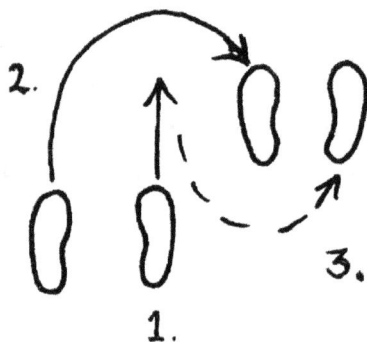

Hexameter with E Crossing: Long   - short   - short
                             1 right foot 2 left foot   3 right foot

Step forwards with the right leg, the left leg crosses over, bring the right leg together next to the left leg.

Step forwards with the left leg, the right leg crosses over, bring the left leg together next to the right leg.

5. Speaking hexameters

"Over the mountains aloft,
came a rush and a roll and a roaring"
                    —from *Andromeda*, Charles Kingsley

a) speak loudly

b) speak softly

c) whispering

d) only in thought

e) then speak in a normal voice

One should have the children read hexameter: (*Hermann and Dorothea* by Goethe). At first read along quietly with the child, then gradually speak more and more softly until the child reads alone. The hexameter can help most illnesses.

6. Vowels *(with jumps)*

7. Rod or ball throwing *(child throws rod or ball while speaking one-syllable word)*

Throw the ball against the wall but catch it again (crack, air, light).

8. Rhythmic R

9. Incarnating and excarnating spirals

Notes from Dr. zur Linden, *Erfahrungsheilkunde*, 1967: Imitation, due to nervousness within the environment, shock. Psychological causes come to the fore with stutterers. The seasons, especially the winters, affect stutterers. Other reasons can be anaemia, exhaustion, infectious diseases, and lack of sleep. A vegetarian diet is better for stutterers than one with meat. Build the self-confidence of the stutterer. Don't simply help the stutterer to overcome his obstacles but rather remain quiet and patient to allow him to find the word by himself. Show the stutterer that you are fond of him and praise him.

XI. Learning Difficulties, Especially Dyslexia and Dyscalculia

With dyslexia, the motor development (reflexes, symmetry, coordination) has been hindered or disturbed. There can be at least five reasons for this.

1. Physical causes

- The ears should be checked regularly. If there is an inflammation of the middle ear in the left ear, the child will be somewhat deaf in the left ear and spatial orientation will be one-sided.

- The child should be examined for anaemia.

- Eczema: (Often such children can't sleep and therefore are not fit for lessons on the following day.)

- Have the children's eyes examined for short or far-sightedness: such children often cannot properly see the teacher, the blackboard, nor their surroundings.

2. Psychological causes

- These children have too little ability to think in the abstract: (the picture of a bear will never become the consonant B for them. They cannot do fractions in mathematics. In order to strengthen their ability to think in the abstract these children need extra lessons and learn by practising more often. Such children learn to read in 5th grade. The class teacher must especially protect such a child from being teased.

- Those children with too strong an ability to think in the abstract cannot bring their imaginative forces into play.

3. Excessive temperaments

A child's temperament must be brought into harmony between the ages of 7 and 14 through the following: seat the children according to their temperaments; do form drawing for the various temperaments; sing songs for the different temperaments: (e.g. a marching song for the choleric, a lullaby for the melancholic).

4. Children in shock

(e.g., due to separation or divorce of the parents, or due to seeing a shocking accident such as the grandfather dying of a heart attack in the child's presence) They can't handle challenge and therefore give up on learning. If the child says too often, "I can't" then one must call in a doctor or the appropriate professional. Such children have a constitution similar to that of hysteric children. Their skin is etherically filled with holes. Such children have wounds in their etheric bodies (trauma) and are often bed-wetters. They frequently have eyes that shine too much. There is always a restlessness around such children.

Game therapy: tell stories (pedagogically-related stories or create a play where you have to enact the roles in stages (acts) as though they were the situations which lead up to the trauma.) When writing: the teacher should guide the hand of the child for a time (the teacher's ego flows to the child and strengthens the child).

5. Late developers, partially handicapped children and children with dyslexia

These children do well in mathematics but can't read or write. Their spatial orientation is often weak, their organ of balance being damaged in such a way that the relationship between right and left is affected. Such children have often as babies left out the "crawling phase." Late developers may have large heads, but not always. One should give these children time and then, all of a sudden, to everyone's surprise, they learn overnight.

See: *Meditativ erarbeitete Menschenkunde* (Rudolf Steiner, 3rd lecture)

Learning Difficulties

Children with learning difficulties think in pictures, not in abstractions. One must lead them by way of imaginations or by doing into the form or into the abstract thought. Such children hear the sounds or tones one after the other: first with the one ear and then shortly thereafter with the other ear. This is also so with their sight. The field of vision for such children cannot cross as is normal. They can't bring the right and left to cross (over) each other. They are light-footed. (Liesbeth van Vewen, therapeutic eurythmist)

These children are often physically too heavy in their limbs. They are inaccurate in their speech. They often have very beautiful, symmetric faces which are, however, a bit wide (rather wide nostrils). The teeth have spaces between them. Their faces are often unformed. The upper organism with its forming powers hasn't penetrated the entire body. Dyslexia appeared for the first time in England in 1905, then in Stockholm, Sweden and then in Cologne, Germany.

The following factors may lead to dyslexia: optic and acoustic effects; an inharmonious family life / a broken home; moving home too often; changing countries; clogged ears or an infection of the middle ear. Children with dyslexia often cannot remember long sentences, due to previous ear problems.

In such cases it may be helpful to have these children read short paragraphs and then retell what they have just read. One must have all of their senses examined by a medical doctor in order to find the origin of the dyslexia. These children cannot cross their arms (E); the ego doesn't penetrate into the etheric.

Jean Lynch, a therapeutic eurythmist: "Children with dyslexia look very young and have difficulties which lie between the physical and etheric bodies. They have to work very hard to get out of the spherical consciousness of the young child and into a linear consciousness, i.e. out of the spherical etheric forces which build the body and into a clear consciousness. They slip back again and again. One must strengthen the forces of their will and the rhythmical forces in order to strengthen the necessary swing in their handwriting. Without a sense of rhythm, these children won't understand what they read or write. One must study all the movements of these children: walking, running, jumping (when 4 years old), skipping (when 7 years old). Children who have dyslexia have great difficulties with their feet. Observe as well, if they make unnecessary secondary movements and if they can do various movements with their feet or with their hands. Such children walk with large, stiff steps. In order to allow them to feel their legs, let them slide on their knees through the room."

Tests for Learning Difficulties (Dyslexia)

Test 1

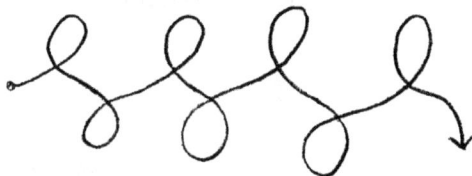

Mesker Therapy: Let the child carry on with this form using his/her finger. (The child moves the first part of the form and then in standing continues the dotted line form with his/her finger, which the therapist guides.)

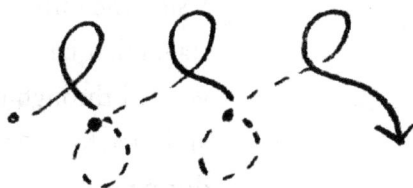

Test 2   *Three phases of hand and arm movements*

Phase 1:
Children under four years of age: If the right hand is contracting into a fist, the other is opening up. This must stop after the age of four. If this doesn't stop, then later on one has learning difficulties with numbers, writing and reading. A part of the etheric within the head becomes free, as it should, when this exercise is stopped.

Phase 2:
Symmetry-phase: If the right hand moves to grasp something, while the left hand moves to grasp it as well. This phase takes place between the ages of five and six, after which time it comes to an end. The etheric partially frees itself from the rhythmic system.

Phase 3:

Lateralization: The one hand does something while the other hand remains still. This begins between the ages of six and eight and continues for the rest of one's life. The etheric body partially frees itself from the metabolic-limb system.

Test 3

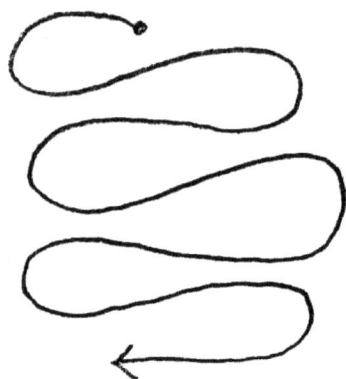

This movement is almost like the back and forth swaying movement in crawling.

Using the form shown, one corrects stages that had not been properly worked through in early childhood and therefore can cause difficulties during puberty.

Dyslexia has a genetic dimension, as well. It is also sometimes connected to illnesses of the immune system.

General Exercises for Dyslexia

1. Knee sliding

Have the children move around the room on their knees to have them free their legs. They usually run with large stiff steps.

2. Contraction and expansion

To harmonize the relationship between the physical and the etheric bodies:

The sun is in my heart
He warms me with his power,
And wakens life and love,
In bird and beast and flower.

The stars above my head
Are shining in my mind,
As spirits of the world
That in my thoughts I find.

The earth whereon I tread
Lets not my feet go through,
But strongly doth uphold
The weight of deeds I do.

Then I must thankful be
That man on earth I dwell,
To know and live the world
 And work all creatures well.

(Alfred Cecil Harwood)

or:

Praise we the sun
His rays warming
His light unfolding
Creative power in me.

(Rudolf Steiner)

3. Steering forwards and behind the back

"I will build me a boat for my sailing
over beautiful billowing sea
it will be my a boat till the sunset
Brings my boat into harbour for me."

4. Hexameter on the Harmonious Eight

5. Anapest

∪ ∪ —— ∪ ∪ —— ∪ ∪ —— ∪ ∪ ——

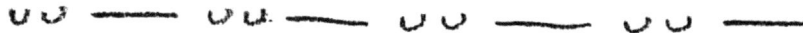

short - short - long,   short - short - long,   short - short - long, etc.

a) clapping and letting the child run in the above rhythm, then he/she must stop abruptly at the sound of a gong

b) begin very slowly, and then get faster and then stop abruptly

c) in all four spatial directions in the room

d) with various rhythms

6. Spatial forms

Preparatory exercise with copper balls.

The copper ball leads the form:

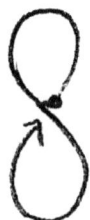

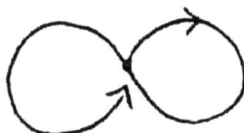

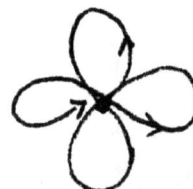

Short – short – long

a. run on the short – short
   stand on the long

b. run on the long
   stand on the short – short

giving the copper ball on the longs

Rhythmic exercise

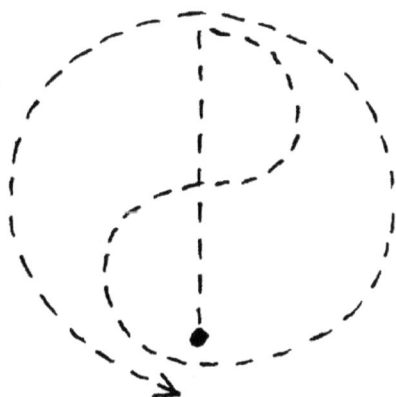

from The Flow

Deep in green woodland's night
Is a brook running light
Flows from hillside to valley a-mumbling,
And the flowers, so fair
Stand amazed as they stare
At the children so happ'ly a-tumbling.

—R. Reinick (for original German, see
Appendices p. 199)

Three-fold Walking:

With the carrying, contract the toes of the feet. With the placing, let them open out (this alters between holding back and letting go)

7. Staircase exercise

E – long – E (upwards)

E – long – E (in the middle)

E – long – E (behind)

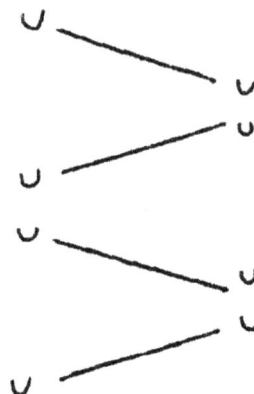

Dyslexic children fall into the weight of gravity and are physically stiff because their etheric forces don't properly penetrate their physical bodies. In this case all rhythmical movements help. Rhythmic repetitions strengthen the etheric. All possible concentration exercises are important, also A and E. All rod exercises help these children to incarnate and strengthen their spatial orientation.

8. Concentration exercise *(fast! no pausing in between)*

forwards: 1 step

backwards: 1, 2 steps

forwards: 1, 2, 3 steps

backwards: 1, 2, 3, 4 steps

forwards: 1, 2, 3, 4, 5 steps

backwards: 1, 2, 3, 4, 5, 6, steps

forwards: 1, 2, 3,4, 5, 6, 7 steps   and variations.

9. Forms — straight and curved *(to strengthen the etheric body)*

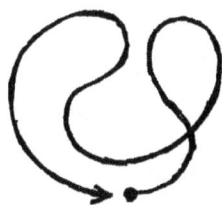

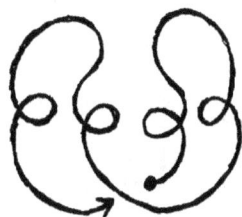

a) Simple, and

b) more complex forms

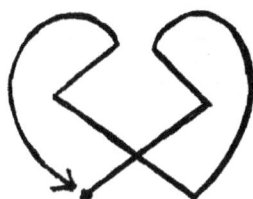

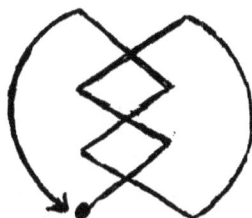

a) Simple, and

b) more complex forms

10. Mirror image forms

Teacher

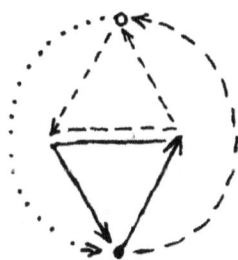

Child

11. Forms with triangles and their mirror-images

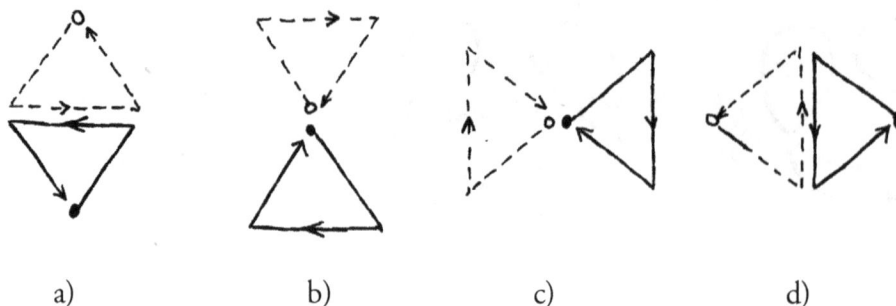

a)   b)   c)   d)

12. Form drawing for stiff joints

Progress from large round forms
to small forms.

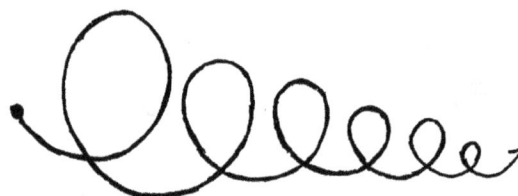

13. Draw or write on the child's back *(then have the child try to guess what has been written or drawn)*

a) geometric forms
b) numbers
c) letters

14. Symmetrical forms

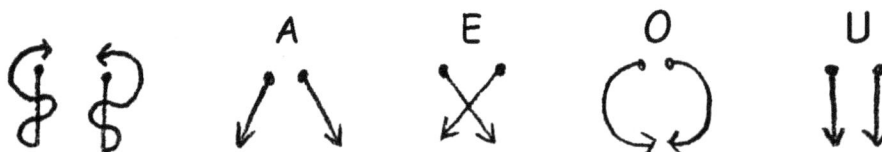

15. Using the directions in space as a basis

Starting from a middle point,

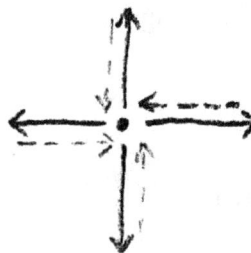

a) Then walking in all directions
and over and again returning
to the middle point.

b)

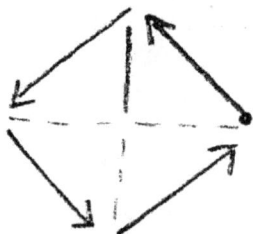

c)

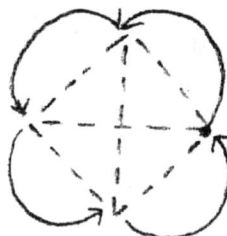

then connecting the four corners   forwards and backwards

d)

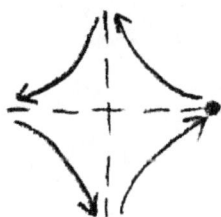

e)

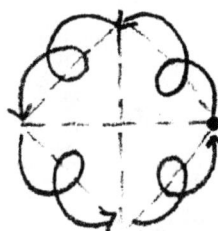

Always do the forms forwards and backwards (4 = the number of incarnation). Doing things in reverse order (Rückschau) strengthens the Ego.

16. Reverse order exercise (Rückschau)

Speaking and moving to texts forwards and backwards.

"Brave and true
I will be,
each good deed
sets me free,
each good thought
makes me strong,
I will fight
for the right
I will conquer
the wrong."

17. "This is S"

18. Evolutionary Sequence with the feet

19. Soul gestures

Love-E
Hope-U
A-Veneration
Yes – No
Sympathy – Antipathy

Consonant Exercises

1. L *(quietly, standing, small, big, small)*

2. L with 1 – 7 – 1

3. M streaming forwards and backwards: *(a low M with the M walking in a rocking step)*

4. Five-pointed star with L and M   *inside ways: M Circle: L*

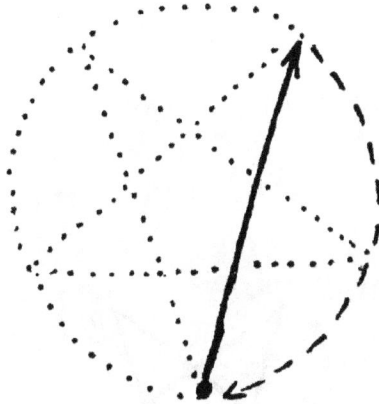

5. Five-pointed star with B and F   inside ways: F Circle: B

6. F forwards and back *(on five-pointed star)*

7. S breathing forwards and back *(on five-pointed star)*

8. S – I

a) in the form
b) with the legs standing

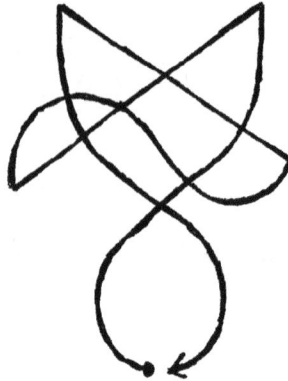

9. N on a five-pointed star *(large in the space, then do the form gradually smaller and smaller, finally very small)*

P

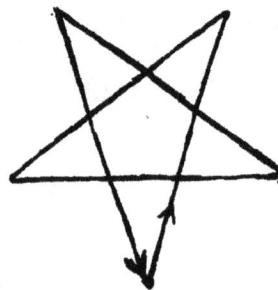

10. L M N R B H S *(with the shoulders)*

a) Triangle Form: Mirror image

11. The four elements

Fire	Earth
F S H C	B P D T G
Sh	K M N

Air	Water
R	L

Distribute the sounds on the four corners of the room.

When the teacher calls out the sound, the child must find the appropriate corner where this sound belongs.

12. Consonant circle

A circle of consonants constructed like a clock so that the child learns the consonants and knows where they are in the circle.

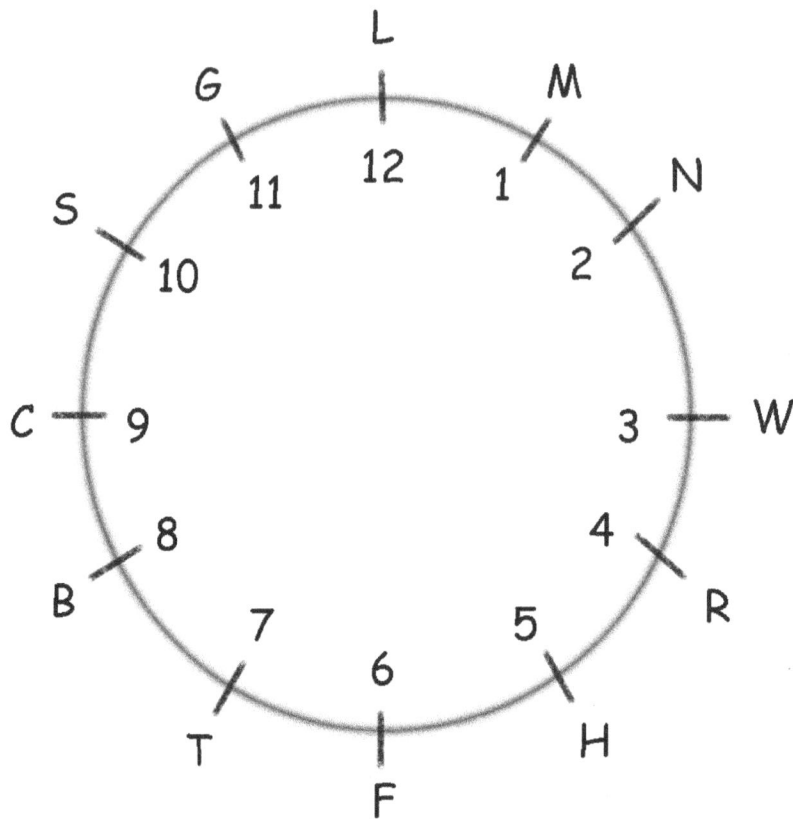

Vowel Exercises

1. Breathing vowels

From small to big to small

2. Moving vowels

A E I O U (to counter the fixed idea: "I can't do it")

3. A Iambic – A trochaic

4. The Big I exercise

5. U – up on the toes and down again (in order to feel their legs)

6. Big E vowel exercise

7. E – over rods (with E stepping over the rods forwards and backwards stepping not jumping)

8. Agility-E

a) striking the elbows on the thighs:

b) in pairs: the partners cross their forearms and hold each other's hands while doing the agility E with their legs.

This helps to get the Ego into the etheric body

9. E – crossing with the feet

short – long – short to the song:

Now show us your feet here,
now show us your shoes,
and watch what the women so busily do....

going to the right:

left foot over right   sideways to the right   left over right

      ∪   —————————————   ∪

going to the left:

right foot over left   sideways to the left   right over left

then once again from the beginning: left crossing over the right.

10. A E I O U: (on a five-pointed star, also in canon)

a e I, o u A, e i O, u a E, i o U
on a five-pointed star also in canon

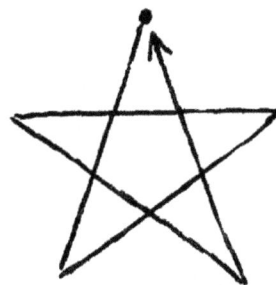

11. Contraction and expansion

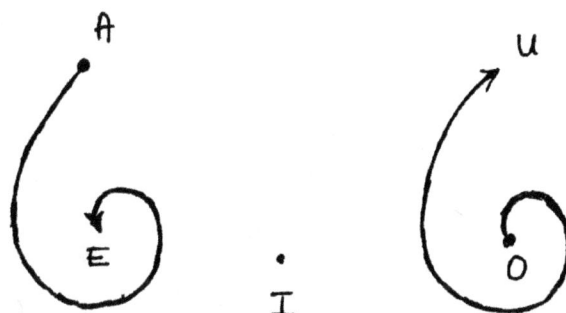

12. I A O (*with a five-pointed star*)

13. I A O

I	A	O
Balance: between right and left	Will: forwards backwards: Destiny	O – Feeling: reveals the human being as soul

14. I A O (*in relation to the directions of space*)

15. A E A - I I A (*the therapist facing the child*)

16. I E I (*on E strike the thigh with the elbow*)

17. Love- E

18. Agility-E

19. A – Veneration

20. I A O to close (to harmonise thinking, feeling, and willing)

Coordination Exercises

1. Stamping and hitting the knees (sitting)

a) hitting both knees with the palms of both hands. Then with the right hand, then left hand (one after the other), then stamping the right foot, then left foot.

b) hit the knee with the palm of the right hand; stamping: right foot, then left foot; then hit the knee with the palm of the left hand

c) hit the right hand on the right knee; stamp with the left foot; stamp with the right foot and hit the left knee with the left hand

2. Anapests

short – short – long	hitting the elbow	(on long)
short – short – long	hitting the shoulders	(on long)
short – short – long	clapping above the head	(on long)
short – short – long	clapping behind the back	(on long)

3. Body geometry

Starting with the arm outstretched with eyes closed, the child must touch the tip of his/her nose with his/her index finger.

4. Straight – curved

Give the child two pieces of chalk,
one in each hand and then let him/her
draw a straight line and a curved form
on the blackboard with both hands
simultaneously:

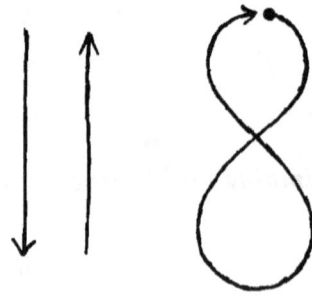

5. Copper rods

Place copper rods on the floor creating a narrow
passage. The child must walk along it, looking straight
ahead and the feet mustn't touch the rods. Have the
child carry a burning candle or a silver bowl filled with
water over this bridge.

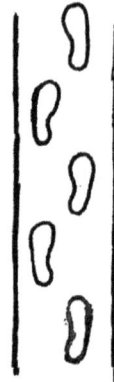

6. Copper rod on the floor

Place one single row of copper rods on the floor.
Cross over the row of rods by crossing the legs
(making an E with the legs)

a) walking forwards and backwards

b) carrying a rod on the head

c) with the rod on the head while walking
   forwards and backwards

d) making E-crossings with the hands
   each crossing with the feet = one E
   crossing with the hands

(This is also good in the 4th grade)

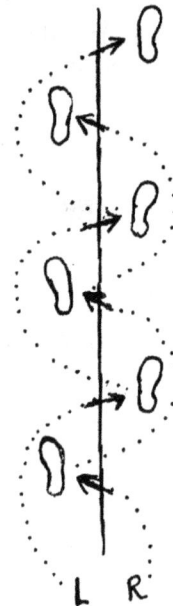

144

7. Throwing beanbags

Fill various little velvet sacks.

Fill one with beans,
another with lentils.
another with split peas.
another with sand.
and one with gravel.

This strengthens the senses of these children: using different colors for the little velvet sacks for the sense of sight, velvet for the sense of touch, and filling the little sacks with different things for the sense of hearing. When one tosses the sacks from one hand to the other, each sack makes a different sound and you can make a small orchestra by doing this.

a) toss the little beanbag in a lemniscate (while standing):

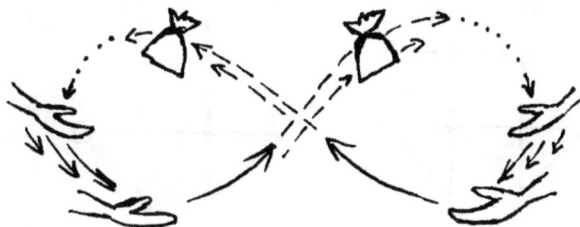

b) Toss a bag in a circle around the body (to develop a feeling for the back).

c) Throw a bag behind one's head while making a crossing by tossing it from the left hand above the head and over to the right hand below.

d) Toss a bag in a large curve (like a rainbow over the head, tossing it from one hand to the other).

e) Two children toss the little bags from the outer hand of the one to the outer hand of the other and vice versa.

Rod Excercises

1. Seven-part Rod Exercise in the space

a) with one step

b) with two steps, and so on

c) moving spatially, freely moving

d) also in mirror-image

2. Seven-part Rod Exercise on this form *(from Höller)*

a)

b)

c)

d)

Change direction at the corners so the starting points are always different.

e) in rhythm: short – short – long – standing and clapping

f) counter-rhythm with the feet: long – short – short

3. *Twelve-part rod exercise*

a) classic, standing
b) on a lemniscate

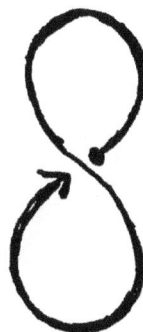

4. *Twelve -part rod exercise (from Höller)*

a) as long as the rod is in front, walk forwards (until the count of 5) on 6 walk backwards and on 11 walk forwards

b) not minding whether the rod is in front or in back:
   from 1–6 walking forwards and from 7–12 walking backwards

5. *Spirals*

a) in standing
b) doing spiral forms spatially   c) spirals on a cross form

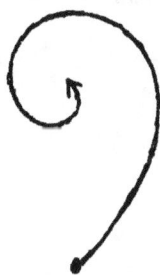 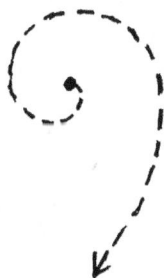 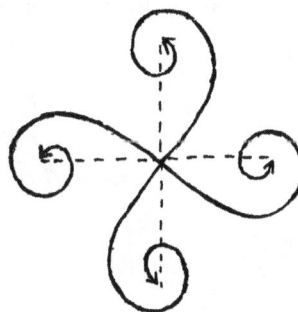

6. Waterfall

a) in standing

b) on a straight I line

7. Qui, Qui

a) classic

b) on a zig-zag form for agility in the fingers and feet

8. Rod throwing

a) short – long, with a jump on the long

b) short – short - long

9. Lemniscate

a) in standing while drawing the form in the air with the rod

b) then while moving on the form of a lemniscate

c) then in standing once again

d) then while only imagining yourself moving along the lemniscate while standing

10. Rolling a copper rod up and down the arms

This helps a child become more aware of his arms.

XII. Left-handedness

Through therapeutic eurythmic exercises, the one-sidedness of the right or left can be developed to a dominance of the one or the other. In the case of cross-dominance and the question of learning to write with the right hand, it is necessary to cooperate with the parents and teachers. (See also Goebel-Glöckner, *Kindersprechstunde*, Stuttgart 2006)

Try to correct only those children with a cross dominance who are between four and nine years old, not older (Dr. Karl König).

It is especially important for these children to cherish their teacher. Allow them to write only as a reward but then with the right hand.

Writing is an activity of the etheric body (habits). The etheric body is stronger on the right than on the left in relationship to the physical. The sound E (eh) fixes the ego in the etheric. In relationship to the astral body, the etheric body is stronger on the left and the astral body is stronger on the right.

Characteristics of left-handed people: weak, nervous, constantly freezing.

Test for left-handedness

have the person:

– cut something
– look through a hole in a piece of paper
– throw a ball
– hammer a nail
– catch a ring (which arm does s/he catch with?)
– walk (which leg does he/she start with?)

Exercises for Lefthanders

1. I A O

With the fingers: begin with the right hand, have them practise it often, only using the left once in a while to balance it out.

2. Vowels

First form half the vowel, always beginning with the right arm and completing it with the left. Then do it with both arms.

3. Evolutionary Sequence

As above with the vowels: first with the right arm, then completing the consonant with the left, then with both arms simultaneously.

4. Agility-E

5. Big E vowel exercise

6. Consonant and vowel exercise *(from Höller)*

Consonants to the right, vowels more to the left

a) right	M	b) right	F	c) right	K
left	O	left	I	left	O
right	M	right	F	right	K
L with both arms		L with both arms		L with both arms	

150

7. An indication of Rudolf Steiner's to a Waldorf teacher *(Karl Schubert)*

With the right foot I will walk it:
(going forwards with one step while right arm makes an I in front)

With the left foot I will leave it:
(going backwards while the left arm does an I downwards and behind)

With the right hand I will fight:
(going forwards, I with the right arm in front above)

With the left hand I will carry:
(walking backwards, the left arm with a carrying gesture)

8. Leg consciousness *(Take steps then suddenly stamp to the right or hop on the right leg.)*

9. Leg-arm consciousness

Jumping on the left leg with the right arm stretched out horizontally and the right leg stretched out in the air parallel to the arm. (See M. Kirchner-Bockholt, *Fundamentals of Curative Eurythmy,* Floris Books, Edinburgh, 2004)

10. Comes a little mouse and builds a little house *(from Rudolf Steiner)*

With the right arm at breast height bent downwards, the child looks down the right arm and up again. Then stretch the arm in I. Do the whole 3 times.

11. An exercise from Rudolf Steiner

Bend the right arm at the chest, then stretch forwards strongly into an I at shoulder height. The right heel as in "agility E," hits the knee of the left leg. Then stretching the arm forwards in an I. In between a step and then repeat from the beginning but not more than eight times. This is a very strenuous exercise.

"Lefthanders must be made dexterous." (Rudolf Steiner)

12. Run with the right arm outstretched

also in the following way:

Stepping over stepping stones
1 2 3,
stepping over stepping stones,
come with me.

The water is deep,
the water is wide,
we jump across
and reach the other side.

13. Verse

A sailor went to sea sea sea

(salute to the right to the
"sea sea sea" stretched up
to the right I)

to see what he could see see see
But all that he could see see see
Was the bottom of the deep blue
sea sea sea

(forward, horizontal I)
(slightly down: 45° I)
(right arm stretched down I)
(only use right arm throughout)

14. Leg-arm exercise

I – fling out the right arm   – 3 x
I – fling out the right leg,   – 3 x
arm and leg together   – 3 x
(finally very loosely as in the shaking L)

15. Musical beat

2/4 beat right – left
(with the arms as well: a strong widening gesture with the right, and bringing in the left as in a contraction.)

16. O – I to the rhythm short – long

left right
O   I

The call of God our Father's sound ...

—J. W. Goethe (see Appendices p. 197 for poem and original German version)

17. Exercise for lefthanders from Ruth Wolf (from an indication by Rudolf Steiner)

Fling the right arm upwards and outwards, left foot steps forward, right leg jumps forward and lands on right foot. With the left arm behind the back, the right arm (makes a turning movement outwards from underneath) relaxed but outstretched (relaxed at the elbow). Then stretching the arm forwards and upwards only until the height of the eyes. Then look along the arm.

18. Rod exercise

Two little rods, one in each hand: with the right little rod over the left arm, stroke as the rod rolls from the shoulder to the hand with the words:

"The left is receiving ..."	With the right little rod tenderly touching the left one (slow)
"The right is achieving!"	The right little rod hits the left one fasr, "The left rests, the right fights." (fast)

19. Jump exercise

Pease porridge hot,
pease porridge cold,
pease porridge in the pot
nine days old …

One stands with the feet slightly apart and the right foot in front. Then one jumps around in the rhythm and always stresses by jumping forwards on the right foot. One begins each line with the right foot in front. On the third line one hops twice on the same foot.

20. Lemniscates (from small to large and small again with the right hand in front of the right side of the chest)

The knight, he slings	8 small	The snap, it slaps
The knight, he springs	8 larger	The snap, it taps
The horse he bites	8 largest	The scissor bites
The rider fights.	(flinging out the arm)	The yarn is nice.
Strongly fighting	8 large	Longest ribbon
Very knightly	8 small	Lazy women
Always dreaming	8 smaller	Shortest ribbon
Knightly seeming	8 smallest	Busy women
		(sew the snap on again)

21. Copper ball exercise

Go around your body clockwise like in the "spiral" rod exercise using a ball or a copper ball (eventually grab the ball more strongly with the right hand and stamp with the right foot).

22. Copper ball exercise

Hickory dickory dock
The mouse ran up the clock
The clock struck one
The mouse ran down
Hickory dickory dock

The ball is in the right hand. On "hickory," in the left hand. On "dickory" place it in your own right hand. On "dock" knock strongly on the left hand of the neighbor to your right. On "the mouse ran up the clock" change ball quickly from one hand to the other on tip-toes. On "the clock struck one," toss the ball into the air. On "the mouse ran down," quickly let the ball fall into the other hand along the symmetry line as one goes into the knees. Then repeat as above for "hickory dickory dock."

23. Copper ball exercise *(counting from 1 to 7)*

– The ball is in the left hand. On 1 place it from your left into your own right hand. Then along a circle (composed of a few people)in front and to the right pass it on.

– Then count 1,2: on 1, place the ball from the left into the right hand and on 2, place it from the right into your own left hand. In the pause, put it behind your back and then place it in the left hand of the neighbour to your right.

– On the even numbers the ball goes behind your back from the left to the right. On the uneven numbers one gives the ball on to the other while moving over the front and to the right.

24. Catch the beanbag

Place a small board on top of a rounded piece of wood making a small seesaw. Place a beanbag onto the board on the side which is touching the ground. Then jump onto that side of the board which is up in the air. This makes the beanbag fly through the air. Catch the beanbag with the right hand. This exercise calls for a lot of skill.

25. Catch and throw the veil

Very playfully activate the direction from left to right as in a game. (This strengthens the flow of the physical stream of movement.) The therapeutic eurythmist tosses a small veil through the air and the child must catch it, preferably with the right hand. If the child catches it with his left hand, give it to him in his right hand. Have the child toss it to the therapeutic eurythmist with a curve over the right.

26. Playful right-sided movements

Crumple a small silk scarf with your hands and place it on the child's head as a hat or a crown and have him hold a rod in his left hand. Then have the child ride to the castle, stop in front of the princess's window, take off the hat and bow or curtsey. While riding away, waving with the little scarf. Do everything as playful right-sided movements.

27. Rod exercises for lefthanders

a) 7-part rod exercise   (right 2x)

b) 7-part rod exercise (variation from Höller): when one goes to the right always make a stamping step forwards; otherwise pull the feet together and stand.

c) Spiral rod exercise (from Höller):

   Only in the lower zone. The right hand grasps the rod strongly and take a stamping step. The left hand takes the rod gently from the right.

Follow your nose along this form

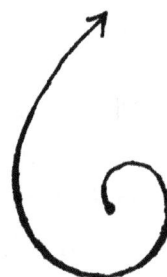

156

d) Turning-throw: (do more often with the right hand than with the left)

e) Throwing and catching:
   – Holding the rod horizontally, toss it upwards, catch it up above
   – Holding the rod horizontally let it fall from above and catch it from underneath
   – Increasing the throwing distance to short – short - long

f) "This is S": (more with the right hand; also on a circle)

g) Run with the rod in the right hand and then touch something with the rod. At first in front, then somewhat more to the right:

h) The child and the therapeutic eurythmist stand across from each other The child throws the rod to the therapist with his right arm while taking a step forwards with the right foot. Then he lowers his right arm in an I, and the left foot is brought up to the right. The therapeutic eurythmist gives the patient the rod. The patient throws the rod again with the right and the exercise begins all over again.

28. Libra gesture *(Libra gesture – C upwards – Libra gesture)*

To encourage a balance so that the right side doesn't get over-strained.

29. L M – L L L M

(For inner balance and as a general harmonizing this is used as a closing exercise and as the culmination for all the exercises for left-handedness.)

XIII. The Formation of the Teeth

"If a four, five or six year old child is clumsy with his arms and hands, and legs and feet, or if it isn't easy to get the child to skillfully perform an action with his arms and legs and even less so with his hands and feet, then one can conclude that the child tends not to be able to take part efficiently in the process of his own teeth-formation. One can especially observe by the way the child moves his arms and hands and his legs and feet symptoms of the same type of child that will most likely turn up later in the process of the formation of the teeth." This process of teeth formation is greatly affected by the very thing that one tries to teach the children preferably early in life: the sense of walking artistically. The child must learn to move his feet artistically while walking. Have him do the Kiebitz jump without M, or something similar so that one foot hits against the other while he walks, or other artistic walking steps. Training the fingers to become skillful (as with needlework) also promotes to a great extent exactly what is involved in the process of the building of the teeth. (Rudolf Steiner, *Spiritual Science and Medicine,* Rudolf Steiner Press, 1975, p. 219; SteinerBooks, *Introducing Anthroposophical Medicine,* 2007)

Too much dancing—of the normal kind—is an example of something that is not so good for the teeth. (Rudolf Steiner, *Spiritual Science and Medicine,* p. 258)

* * *

The forces of thinking are set free with the process of teeth formation. If the thinking forces are not released properly, then this can be seen within the teeth-building process and then the sounds in the therapeutic eurythmy will help. For example, the Apollonian sounds – A and O.

Just as the second set of teeth drive out the baby teeth, so the individual ego pushes away the stream of hereditary.

The incisor teeth:	relate to the nerve-sense system	– thinking
The eyetooth or canine teeth:	relate to the rhythmic system	– feeling
The molars:	relate to the metabolic-limb system	– will

(Rudolf Steiner, *Curative Eurythmy,* Rudolf Steiner Press, London, 1983)

Exercises

1. *"Teeth exercises" L A – L O*

Take hold of the L from down low and bend the knees while doing so. Do not stick out the bottom. Feel the golden character in the hands. Sense the warm formative force in the upper arms, remaining well forwards, then over your head and really turn the palms upwards. Then feel the wings in the entire space behind you. Do all exercises with joy and strength while jumping far forwards with X-legs.

Do O with both arms and both legs. O with the arms over the head or in the middle.

One can do the big A vowel exercise here too.

With the arms

For the teeth in the upper jaw: L L L A

For the teeth in the lower jaw: L L L O

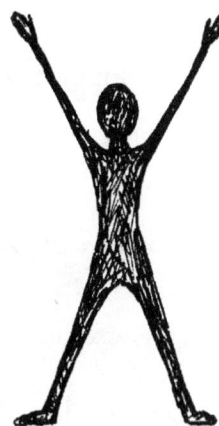

(See *Fundamental Principles of Curative Eurythmy* by Kirchner-Bockholt; Floris Books, Edinborough; 2004)

2. *Rocking-step*

Do first with A and O, in-breathing with A, out-breathing with O.

a) first in standing
b) then, A from above downwards while moving backwards: We have the out-breathing in the A and O (In A is also something of the in-breathing; it has both)

3. L – A L – O *(with the rocking-step)*

L – A backwards, L – O forwards

a) forwards – backwards – forwards: O
b) backwards – forwards – backwards: A
c) forwards – backwards – forwards :

    L   A   O   L A O with the rocking-step

4. The Apollonian sounds

For the upper teeth, stimulate the forming forces; that is, activity from the front going backwards; for the lower teeth, stimulate the activity behind going forwards.

5. All geometrical forms as mirror-image forms

Preparatory exercise:

– I A O in standing, A leaning backwards behind the pillar, and O forwards
– expand backwards, contract forwards – in the middle
– expand backwards, leading into an A, arms downwards; contract forwards, leading into an O – from below returning back

a)

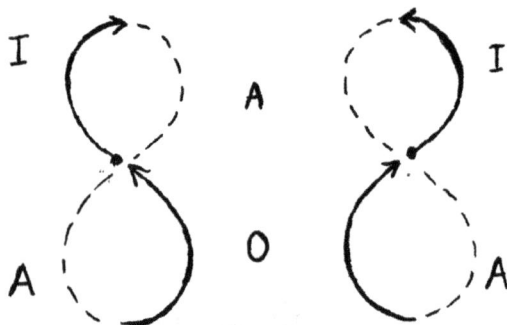

Weaving radiance   I
Strength of weaving   A
Light of strength   A
Lo, This is man   O

—Rudolf Steiner
(see Appendices p. 199 for original German)

b)

I   standing,
A moving from front to back
O moving from back forwards

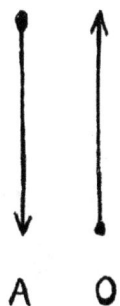

A   O

c)

3 X	*L*	*L*	*L*	*A*	*L*	*L*	*L*	*O*
2 X		*L*	*L*	*A*		*L*	*L*	*O*
1 X			*L*	*A*			*L*	*O*
1 X			*L*	*A*			*L*	*O*
2 X		*L*	*L*	*A*		*L*	*L*	*O*
3 X	*L*	*L*	*L*	*A*	*L*	*L*	*L*	*O*

A standing, leading from above down and behind

O from down to up and forward

d) the same thing on the I – line

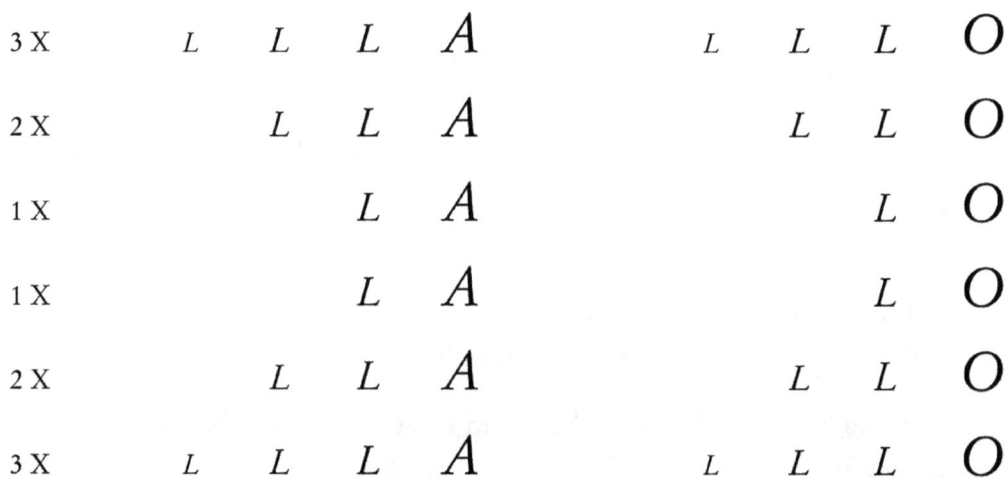

161

6. G *in addition to other sounds* (to activate power of decision)

G L	A		G L	O
in standing,	downwards		standing,	upwards

7. S *in addition to other sounds: (for when the formative forces are missing)*

S L	A		S L	O
standing,	downwards		standing,	upwards

SGL	A		SGL	O
standing,	downwards		standing,	upwards

8. *Dexterity exercises*

a) L with every finger followed by A or O.
   This with the right hand, the left hand and with both hands.

   Children who have problems with their teeth must be taught to become skillful with their fingers.

b) Sideways "Kiebitz" jumps for agility (Lili Herz, therapeutic eurythmist)

c) Vowels: jumping strongly onto the feet:

   There dances a bee bah booterman
   Around our house and in, diddle doom

d) Agility-E:

Nights on mountains
Dance they quickly
dance the dwarf-men
Laughing silly
quickly, quick!
Resting now.   —H. Diestel (Original German in Appendices p. 200)

e) short – short– long on the castle form:

He who likes much advice
Is late for deeds more than twice.
He who's quick in what he thinks
He will win in two winks.

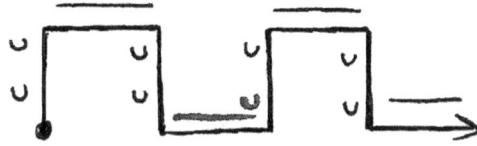

—F. Rückert (Original German in App. p. 212.)

f) Lay 3 copper rods on the ground in front of you. Stand in U behind them.
Rock back and forth between the tip of the toes and the heel.
On "... half past eight," jump over the three rods

Rock rock rockedy rock
wake me up at five o'clock
five o'clock is much too soon
wake me up in the afternoon
afternoon is much too late
wake me up at half past eight.

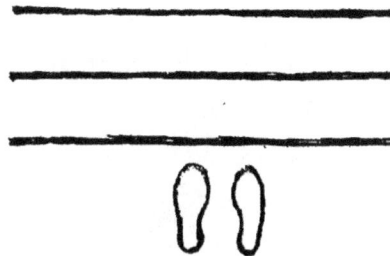

9. Forms with mirror-images

Thinking, feeling and willing are mirrored in the teeth.

a)

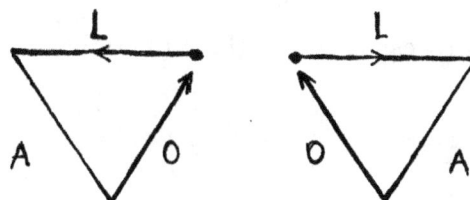

b) 4 x L moving the straight line
    Then strengthen A with B A.

    Then strengthen O with C O.

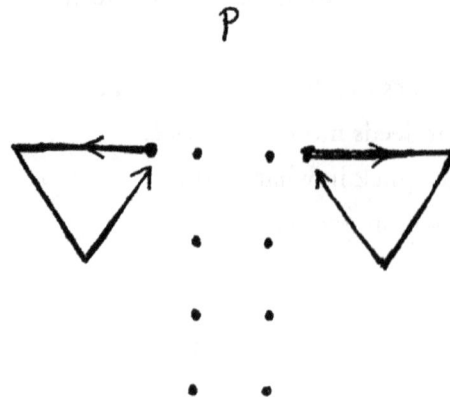

10. Alternating between straight lines and curves to strengthen the etheric

The etheric forces become free for the child's thinking when the adult teeth break through.

If the cutting of the adult teeth and the coming of his second set of teeth happens too irregularly, then one can assume that there is a weakness in the child's etheric body.

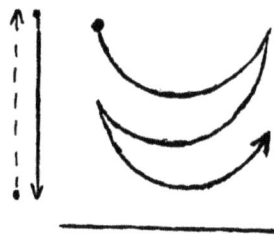

3x L A	3x L O
(Lead A down to mouth height)	(Lead O from below up to mouth height)

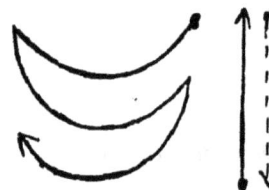

Use symmetrical forms as the teeth are built symmetrically.

11. *L A O O A L*

1. L
2. A
3. O
4. O
5. A
   L standing

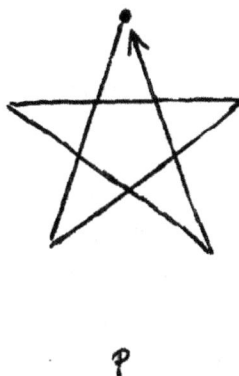

"Doing many speech-formation exercises too helps the children's teeth-formation process."
(Dr. Belarth)

12. *L A - L O (from Linda Nunhofer)*

L 3x with arms and legs (but not with X-jump), then A from above and going deep down and A jump into the legs, L and O 3x from below upwards with an O-jump in the legs

- 3x L forwards, 3x A with a jump back
- 3x L backwards, 3x O with a jump back

13. *Exercises (from Margaret Thiersch)*
(The spine is also related to the teeth and often to a slow digestion.)

- Rhythmical R for the back
- Rocking L in the horizontal
- M if the child squints
- L with X-leg jump going backwards; L with X-leg jump going forwards
- A from above going downwards in standing; O from below going upwards to the middle in standing
 (Always do both L A and L O together because they should work harmoniously with one another.)
 Prepare the X-leg jump by jumping the vowels with the legs

14. LA - LO *(from Dr. Gudrune Hoffmann)*

Do L O many times, O beginning in front of the breastbone but nevertheless build the O from behind towards the front. It must be an O from the beginning of the movement on.

"If one has a protruding jaw then A is used to help correct this animalistic gesture. The lower set of teeth is formed from behind and going forwards: O. The upper set of teeth is formed from in front and going backwards: A." (cf. Rudolf Steiner, *Curative Eurythmy,* Lecture 8, Rudolf Steiner Press, London, 1983)

Rhythm: 1:4 4 x L and 1 vowel

A – breathing out from the head.
A – activates the exhalation and forming power.

15. N

One can also use the N for the process of forming the teeth. ...Just as N works to build and strengthen the bones in the back of the head that have remained too soft. As well, the N can be used prophylactically for the teeth that are becoming damaged. In a good way one can influence the teeth-forming process through training the hands and feet to become skillful and thereby supple so that the soul can stream into the fingers. This happens to a great extent through the N gesture.

(Margarete Kirchner-Bockholt, *Fundamental Principles of Curative Eurythmy,* Floris Books, Edinburgh, 2004)

16. Close with T A O

Exercises for Children with Braces

(even until the age of 12 and 13)

- L with X-jump, big A vowel exercise

- S with O jump

- G with X-jump

- strengthen the rhythmic system

- have then do large forms

- L and M

XIV. Kleptomania

Moral blindness and moral judgment only come to expression within earthly existence. Moral judgment only begins when one must choose between good and evil. For the spiritual world good and evil are simply characteristic qualities. Due to inhibitions in the astral body the kleptomaniac doesn't find access to that which in the outer world is correct balance of judgment among human beings.

Because of the inhibitions the kleptomaniac can't develop his astral body enough to be able to feel a sense for moral judgment. The child doesn't enter the physical world far enough with his astral body. For such a child the concept, "I own something," or "that belongs to someone else" has no meaning at all, nor has he any sense for such judgments. (Rudolf Steiner compares kleptomania to color blindness.)

Such a child vividly experiences finding or discovering something, something surprises or interests the child. But already here the conceptual ability ends: the child's astral body has not penetrated the region of the will but more or less remains in the intellectual sphere. This means that the organs of the will atrophy around the area of the temples. The result is that what is good for the mind gets used in the will. If this applies to the sphere of the intellect then these children become apathetic. If it is taken up in the sphere of the will, they become kleptomaniacs.

Kleptomania is difficult to resist because at this young age when one could fight against it, one hasn't noticed it yet. (Children live in the imitation of their surroundings.) One notices the first inclinations after the child acquires his second teeth but even now the soul is not far enough on the physical plane to develop another sense for moral judgment other than "I like goodness, evil doesn't please me" (only an aesthetic judgment). Here the educator must set an example for the child and the child must have confidence in him.

How Does One Recognize Kleptomania in Early Childhood?

Children who are incredibly joyous and have a special liveliness, develop by means of that which they take a great delight in, that which they have already acquired. Children click with their tongue when they have learnt a new word (a kind of egotism). Around the time the child gets his second teeth this clicking with their tongue changes into a clearly noticeable vanity (which grows out of a greed, and shows itself in that the child dresses purposely different from the norm.)

If such a child grows up in an environment and without borders where he is allowed to do as he pleases, then certain intellectual characteristics slip down into the will area causing kleptomania to appear.

If such a child grows up in an environment where there is a love for order, almost military-like, then perhaps he will go on to study and become skillful. Then he might become, for example, a natural scientist with a great passion for collecting things.

A child stealing sweets doesn't necessarily mean he is a kleptomaniac. They simply are not getting enough sweets at home. The teacher can give the child some honey or some other good sweet in the break. Children who have "small heads" need more sweet foods. The therapeutic eurythmist should also give such a child something sweet to eat. Usually thereafter the stealing of chocolate and candy stops.

How Can One Resist Kleptomania?

1. Some sense of order, strictness and justice.

2. Develop pedagogical stories that have an inner enthusiasm: (e.g. one digs a hole and falls into it himself when he acts like a kleptomaniac). Don't get tired of telling these stories.

3. Medicaments: Injections with Hypophysis cerbri and honey because the temporal lobes are deformed. We should be concerned that these deformations could be influenced by opposing growth forces.

4. Therapeutic Eurythmy: apply it intensively and energetically. Do vowels with the legs.

Exercises

First create the child's own space.

1. Move E on tip toes *(as often each day as possible)*
　　　　　　—Margarete Kirchner-Bockholt, *Principles of Curative Eurythmy*

2. Do vowels with the legs —Margarete Kirchner-Bockholt

3. Hopping vowels with the legs quickly *(find short humorous poems for this)*

a)

```
        A        ↑
 ―――――――E――――――✳―――――――
        A        |
 ―――――――E――――――✳―――――――
        A        |
 ―――――――E――――――✳―――――――
        A        |
 ―――――――E――――――✳―――――――
                 |
```

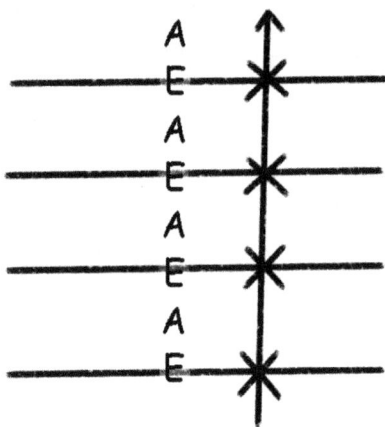

b) A race with the legs crossed in E
   (hold a coin or a ribbon between
   crossed legs)

c) short - short – long over rod rolling
   the rod from the toes onto the heels
   then E-crossing over the rod

d) short – short – long catching rod
   horizontally with E-crossing on the longs

e) alliterations with E-Push between
   child and teacher with arms in E

f) do this twice as fast as well.
   Agility-E with the legs

g) a humorous Poem: Jump fast with the vowels in the feet:

Whether the weather be hot, or whether the weather be not
Whether the weather be cold, or whether the weather be not
We'll weather the weather, whatever the weather
Whether we like it or not.

"... then the intellectual area slips down into that of the will and kleptomania can arise. By practising the vowels using the legs one drives the intellectual out of the will and one drives the efforts that lie within the vowels themselves into the will."

(Rudolf Steiner, *Education for Special Needs,* Rudolf Steiner Press, London, 1996)

4. Kleptomania E

Sitting cross legged with the arms crossed as well so that one can (with the hands) grab hold of the tips of the toes lying parallel to the hands (remain in this position for 10-15 minutes). This exercise should be done over a period of three months.

5. Strengthen the memory by retrospective thinking

a) Speech formation exercises to be done backwards

　e.g., The father reads a book.
　　Book a reads father the.

b) Saying numbers forwards and in reverse order: 3426 – 6243

c) Ask them to talk about things they can imagine from previous years.

6. Sequence of consonants (that have a stimulating effect: L M N P Q)

7. Big A-Exercise to the poem

I saw, I saw
How the sun from afar
Did hold the earth in her arms: ah, ah!

In mothers' eyes
in flowers' sighs

I saw the sun
shining, shining.

} with the swinging part of the exercise

(from original German text by Hedwig Diestel, see Appendices p. 198)

8. First child lesson with Ilse Rolofs

When she takes on a child, she has the child:

a) walk while doing an A eurythmically with his arms

b) walk a five-pointed star

c) speak the morning verse or his own personal poem and write it out to see how his handwriting looks

d) walk a lemniscate with his eyes closed

e) look at the child's physical characteristics and proportions: (large head, small head, hair color, feet, etc.)

Then in the evening observe the child inwards spiritually and above all imagine to oneself how the child would look if he were healthy. Then work out exercises for the child.

For seven weeks Mrs. Rolofs does the same exercises daily. Either one takes the school vacation as the pause or one takes a break for two to three weeks. During the break the exercises can take hold and can inwardly strengthen the child.

Rudolf Steiner said that if one constantly practises with children without ever taking a break then the exercises can easily work in the opposite way or even be harmful!

At the end of the seven week period Mrs. Rolofs invited the class teacher and the subject teachers and presented a kind of therapeutic eurythmy festival. By doing this the teachers gradually developed a sense for therapeutic eurythmy.

XV. Autism

"Mental illness is the only illness in which the physical body is actually useless. The organic disorders are so irreversible that the ego can no longer connect itself with the physical body." (Rudolf Steiner)

Autism sets in after the age of two. Some children begin to regress in their development at the age of three, in such cases the ego simply withdraws. At three years old some children begin to recede in their development; the ego withdraws. If these children are too aware too soon (perhaps even during pregnancy) their sheaths are ripped apart and the child's ego itself withdraws and may be far away. These children are like a crystal. They also have a strong relationship to the mineral kingdom. The ego cannot take hold of the sheaths and therefore these children lose the ability to imitate.

Very often these children have very intellectual parents. The mother, for example, may be a chemist and not have time for her children. The mother maybe too bound to her child (like a symbiosis). There also could be pre-birth causes. The ego can withdraw even during the pregnancy.

In autism the four upper senses (Hearing – Word – Thought – Ego) cannot grip into the body properly. The four lower senses (Touch – Life – Movement – Balance) do not function well, especially not the sense of touch. Autistic children must be brought in from the periphery, for example, by stroking.

Exercises

The therapeutic eurythmist can have a little dwarf that always greets the child and watches, so that there is not such a direct contact between the eurythmist and the child.

1. Running movement *(take the child by the hand and run into the room)*

"Run my horsey, run my horsey,
Run real fast towards home you go:
I and you, I and you."

a) on "I" one touches one's own chest; on "you" reach out towards the other in U.

b) on "Run real fast towards home you go," hold hands and dance around in a circle.

2. Body geography *(one mainly works with the sense of touch)*

I have two feet with which to greet the earth.
I have eyes, a nose and a mouth,
and I can feel all the way down to the ground   (down to the ground with
Two hands as well, oh joy! They are quite skillful people.   the whole body)
In daylight they can take a walk, at night they can't be seen at all.   (hands behind back)

3. Verse

Little ball now you must wander   (Pass a little copper ball along the form of
From the one hand into the other   a lemniscate into the child's hand.)
Oh how nice, oh how nice

And my ball cannot be seen.   (While holding the ball, turn or twist the
                                          wrist back and forth. Do this with each
                                          hand and with the ankles.)

4. Child and Therapist with copper balls

The child holds two copper balls and sits on the floor across from the therapist, who takes the child's wrist and guides the child's arms in a kind of contraction/expansion-like movement. In the contraction which takes place at the middle of the symmetry-line, both copper balls hit and ring out: "an experience of the ego-line."

5. B: with the feet *(building a castle around a copper ball)*

a) at first a small B

b) then a larger B

c) then look to see if a king, a queen or a princess would be able to live in the space created.

6. R with a thick copper foot roller *(stimulates the child's own movement)*

Ride to the castle with:

"Ree rah roach, we're riding in the coach,
we're riding in the carriage,
ree rah roach!"

The therapeutic eurythmist and the child stand across from each other. They do an R together and on "we're riding in the coach," they go with strong steps to the castle. R going forwards and backwards (ego-line). This exercise needs a big thick copper roller.

7. Interval of the fifth *(downwards)*

The child stands in front of the therapeutic eurythmist with her back to the therapist and listens to the descending musical intervals of fifths coming from behind her. The therapeutic eurythmist plays a cantela, a children's harp or lyre and repeats a descending interval of the fifth. The I of the child sinks into the child through these fifths.

8. *A E I*

The therapeutic eurythmist stands behind the child and guides his arms:

In the castle of gold, in the castle of gold	A A
There is so much to see	E
The king and the dear queen are there	I I
And walk through the gates of gold.	G
On her throne of gold the princess sits:	O in the middle sphere
And listens to the tolling bell,	L L L
She wears like the sky a robe of blue	B B
With glitter glittering stars upon.	(laughing fingers)

9. *The Prince*

"Now the prince to the castle rides
on the horse sits the knight up on high."

Autistic children love humorous things.

∪ ∪ ⎯⎯⎯⎯⎯⎯

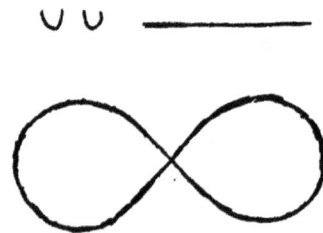

10. *Stimulating rhythm* (Short – short – long)

11. *The Wedding Dance*

Take the child by both hands dancing around in a circle

"Cling, clang Gloria, marries in the castle
Cling, clang Gloria, marries in the castle."

Preparatory exercise before the story

Autistic children love to sit on the therapist's lap. The lyre is played to sound as if the wind were blowing and then when she stops playing she speaks the breath consonants (because these children are often tense): F V. She H.

These exercises can be used as preparatory exercises before combining various exercises to construct an entire story, which can stimulate the senses. The therapist can try to reactivate the ego by way of the 12 senses:

– Body geography (the sense of touch on one's own body)

– The sense of touch on the hands and feet (a lemniscate with a copper ball in the palm of the hand while walking the lemniscate). B – with the feet (Build a castle around a copper ball while sitting on the floor.) Also: "A bird comes flying."

– Creating a middle line when the copper balls hit together: symmetry

– Stand up, holding a copper foot roller and with R. (on the ego-line) ride to the castle. (stimulates the sense of one's own movement)

– Listen to the little golden bell tone of the castle bell. (Build a new sheath around the child with the gesture for the interval of the fifth.)

– After the interval of the fifth, it is possible to do the sound for incarnating: A. The therapeutic eurythmist stands behind the child and guides his arms in A A I I T. (These sounds speak to the ego.)

– Then O: the princess speaks: The therapeutic eurythmist doesn't do the sound U of Old Saturn because she wants to lead the child out of the realm of Saturn.

– Then L L and B B and Laughter: with the fingers like little glittering stars

– Anapest rhythm (short – short - long): the prince rides to the castle on a lemniscate form. "Knock, knock, knock open the gate !" (to wake up the princess)

– This is the most important moment in the entire sequence. The child and the therapeutic eurythmist stand across from each other. They look at one another. This is an important moment since up until now the therapeutic eurythmist has stood either behind or next to the child. Now they look at one another. The child can have a sense of himself!

– Both the child and the therapeutic eurythmist hold each other's hands and dance the "Wedding Dance" going around in a circle.

These children especially love certain words like "the sound of the little bell."

One child's name was "Michael." He called himself "Uncle Meesh." One day he said, "Onkel Mich, Onkel Mich, das bin Ich!" (das bin Ich = that's me). Such moments are important for the therapeutic eurythmist and the child.

XVI. Sexually Abused Children

The astral body and the ego of the child are "shocked to death," so to speak, and hurled out of the body due to this inhuman deed.

Characteristics

- Limits/uprightness (they know no bounds) : They get under your skin and want you to get under their skin (abuse again). They play mainly in the horizontal. They loll about and are always leaning on others. They come up near to others either too easily or else keep themselves very closed off.

- Manipulation: These children need to be allowed to determine what they want to do. They need a sense of security on the one hand and on the other hand they evade or avoid situations.

- Circulation: Their warmth does not reach into the periphery and their breathing is too shallow. They don't live in their own house (body) and are stuck in the head realm. These children do not want to go into their own "house" (body) because it is soiled. Give them the feeling that one can clean this house, and that it is a beautiful house in which one may happily live.

- Eating disorders: There is a rejection of sexual maturity in anorexic tendencies. There can also, however, be bulimia (sexually abused women are corpulent between their hips and thighs: the damaged area is "bundled up"). By over-eating one cuts oneself off from one's surroundings (one's sense of taste is constantly being stimulated in order not to live in one's house/body or in order to keep sexual stimulation in check.). They over-eat in order to reduce the attraction of being a beautiful woman so that no man would want them. (This is very self-aggressive behavior: such women try to tear down their own house.) It is very painful to move into one's own house. Their "house" has been invaded at the wrong moment, and not by oneself but rather by someone else.

– Sleeping disorders: Children are often abused at night. This disturbs the rhythm by which the ego normally excarnates while sleeping and incarnates in waking. Abuse can lead to bed-wetting or even to smearing their own excreta everywhere.

– Psychological problems: There is the tendency to remain a victim – to invite renewed abuse or even the tendency to become an abuser oneself, to be cruel to animals or smaller weaker children.

– Speech impediments: stuttering and an unformed speech and baby-talk because one cannot talk about what has happened. Speech and the sexual organs are related to one another. The speech doesn't descend into the deeper adult range because one cannot speak about what has happened.

– Abused children withdraw into a fantasy world. They have multiple split-personalities (schizophrenia). Often they have a childish sexually-inviting type of behavior.

– Abused children often have poor concentration and problems with restlessness. They are never in the center of any room but rather are to be found somewhere on the periphery either in a corner or under a table. In a room they remain at the periphery and cannot stand in the middle. Neither can they come into their own center. They stand on chairs, or hide under desks. It is important to awaken trust, security, love and understanding in abused children.

Exercises

1. Incarnation exercises

Big A vowel exercise
Big E vowel exercise
Big I vowel exercise
Big O vowel exercise
Big U vowel exercise

Begin preferably with U or E

2. B for the kidneys

a) Big A vowel exercise

b) Measuring rhythms: (Taktieren) rhythms: short – short - long
long – short - short
changing rhythms

c) Harmonious Eight with a copper ball

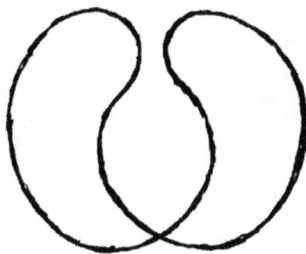

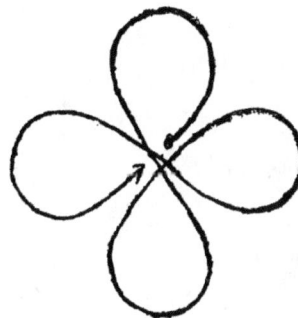

E.g. all forms that will strengthen the center

d) Contraction and expansion:

"In breathing grace may two-fold be
we breath air in, then let it free.
The in-breath binds,
The out unwinds.
Thus with marvels life entwines
Then thanks to God when we are pressed
And thank Him when He grants us rest."

(original German text by J.W. Goethe, Appendices p. 200)

e) Straight and curved lines:

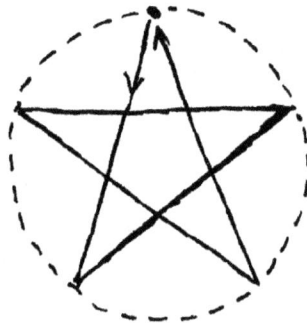

3. Beautiful Poems

E.g. "At the Ringing of the Bells Ring" by Rudolf Steiner

To wonder at beauty,
Stand guard over truth,
Look up to the noble,
Decide on the good:
Leads man on his journey
To goals for his life,
To right in his doing,
To peace in his feeling,
To light in his thought
And teaches him trust,
In the guidance of God
In all that there is:
In the widths of the world,
In the depths of the soul.

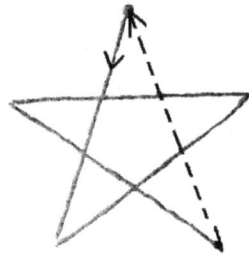

Lines 1 - 4

("breath" on 5th star path)

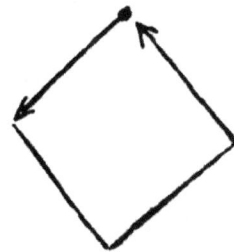

Lines 5 - 8

Line 9: in standing

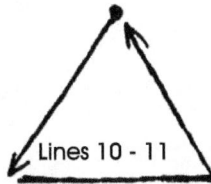

Lines 10 - 11

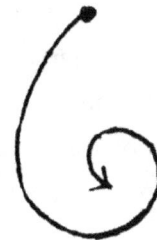

Lines 13 - 14

(translation by Arvia Mackayc Ege;
see Appendices p. 196 for the original German)

With older children, do this with a Rückschau (reverse order).

4. Evolutionary Sequence

Because the evolutionary stream has been interrupted in the child. To be done with the arms, then legs, and finally both arms and legs.

5. "To build a house"

In order to strengthen the harmonic streams in the body and to act against posture problems

a) 7-part rod exercise:

"The earth is firm beneath my feet	(down)
The sun shines bright above	(up)
And here I stand	(right)
So straight	(left)
And strong	(right)
For all to know	(up)
And love."	(down)

"Gainst all violent powers	(down)
Defiance maintaining	(up)
Ne'er bending nor yielding	(bending – right; yielding - left)
Their own strength revealing	(right)
Call out the poor ones	(up)
The gods here to come."	(down)

6. An in-winding spiral

Prepared very slowly, beginning with B

7. *To strengthen the etheric*

a) slowly accelerating – quickly slowing down

b) alternate between straight and curved

c) the entire alphabet

d) A-Veneration Love–E Hope-U
   (one after the other 10 times)

8. *"Bringing the ship of life back to its course"* *(from Mrs. De Jaager)*

A form given to a woman whose life's ship was no longer on course. Do this with children when their life's ship has been blown off course. (with appropriate vowels with or without planets)

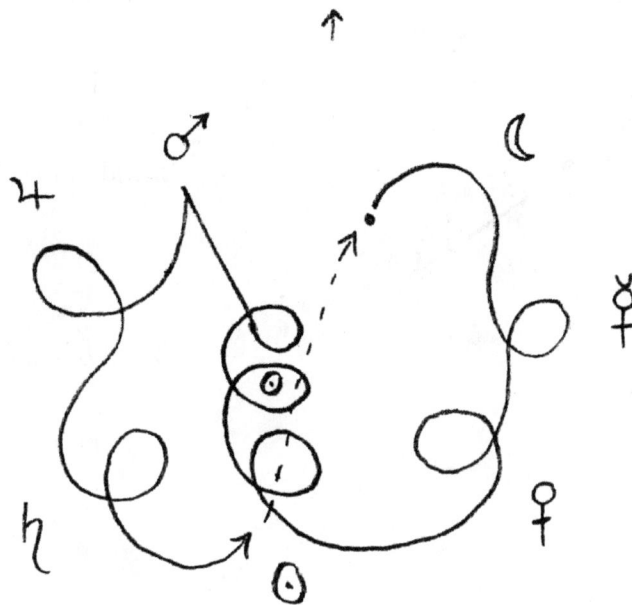

9. Five-Pointed Star and Vowels

The five-pointed star is important for children and teenagers.
Objectivity helps to heal teenagers. Five-pointed star geometry and vowels:

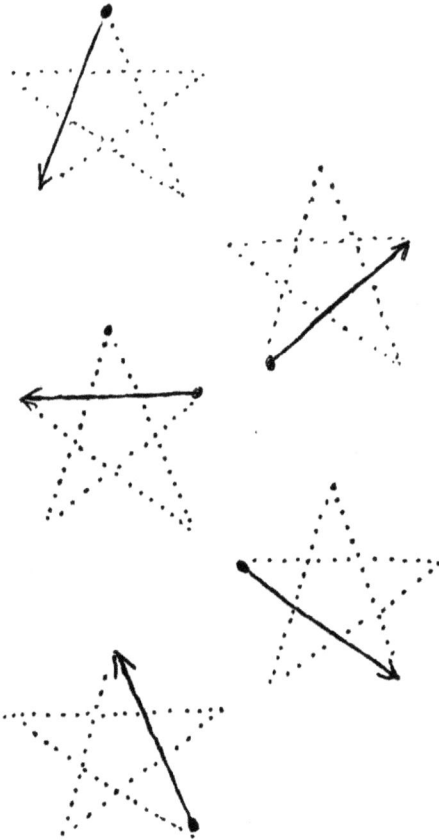

World of angles

A

World of the cross

E

World of the straight

I

World of the circle

O

World of parallels

U

10. From Periphery to Center

The basic direction of movement exercises for people who have been abused is from the periphery towards the center.

– First do large gestures for the vowels, then do the same bringing them into one's heart. Also, do a large five-pointed star, then a smaller five-pointed star: (5 steps, 3 steps, 1 step).

11. Concentration Exercises

12. Rückschau (reverse order) exercises *(done forwards and backwards: with forms, sounds and poems)*

XVII. Blindness

Blind people excarnate easily. They construct their own world. One can guide them into the space around them by means of vowels and consonants.

Exercises

1. First small in the hands

Hands together in U, then open in A, then cross and touch in E, and form a round in O.

2. Building a house

– walls of the house: U on the side of the body:	U
– a roof over the head:	A
– a dome over the head:	O
– windows closed:	E
– windows open:	A
– the human being steps through the door:	I

Through the vowels the human being takes hold of himself from within and takes hold of the space around him!

The consonants work from the outside in, to form the human being.

3. Have the blind child touch objects:

– a soft little velvet pillow:	M
– take a copper ball in the hand and put the fingers well around it:	B
– touch the floor with the palm of the hand, or the therapist's hand:	D
– blow little feathers:	F
– push away a stone with the hands or feet:	G

4. Open the stable door

– A.

– open the door to the stables with A

– then let a little lamb run forwards through the door,

– then, a little mouse going on tiptoes,

– then, have a rabbit or a little dog jump and a heavy bull stamp.

Further recommendations (Trude Thetter)

– Practice many rhythms, tone eurythmy: pitch, beat, etc.

– In order to stop blind people from knocking into people or objects, have them take each other's hand very often so that they get a feeling for the distance between people. They can even try to move along a pentagram.

– Always picture them to yourself as normal human beings and do not draw attention to their blindness. If they can't move forms right away, simply take their arms and lead them around the room.

XVIII. Hydrocephalus Exercises

Exercises

1. Short – Long – Short

(rhythm with the child in the therapist's arms walking sideways and forwards)

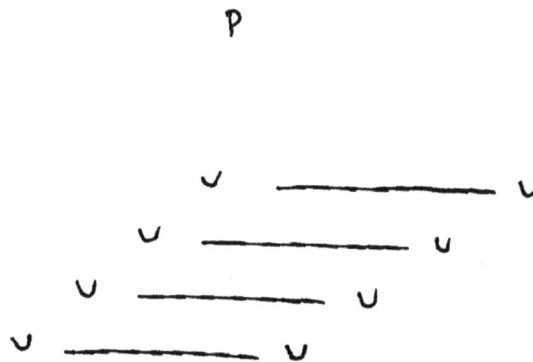

P

ᴗ ——————— ᴗ

ᴗ ——————— ᴗ

ᴗ ——————— ᴗ

ᴗ ——————— ᴗ

2. B gesture around the child

3. O from above going downwards

4. M from above going downwards

5. Singing fifths from up to down

6. Evolutionary sequence: (later on)

7. A and U in the legs

8. Around the head

V A
V E
V I
V O
V U

For little children: singing around the head: "Vigela, vegele"

Tendency to Hydrocephalus (large head)	Tendency to Microcephalus (small head)

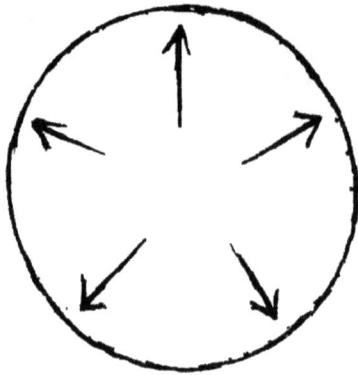

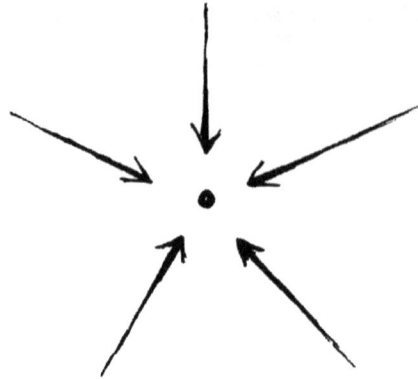

– overpowering metabolic pole

– expansion

– softness (blood)

– generative forces too strong

– embryo period traits retained

– late intellectual development

– strong imagination

– dreamy, not matter-of-fact

– artistic disposition

– sugar process & building-up tendencies

– warmth-sugar-silver

– flowers

– overpowering of the nerve-sense pole

– drawing in

 – hardness (nerves, bones)

– degenerative forces too strong

– premature aging traits

– early intellectuality

– abstract thinking, sober, awake

– matter-of-fact

– little artistic disposition

– salt process and breaking-down tendencies

– coolness-salt-lead

– roots

Appendices

Original Verses and Poems

Kindergebet

Vom Kopf bis zum Fuss
Bin ich Gottes Bild,
Vom Herzen bis in die Hände
Fühl ich Gottes Hauch;
Sprech ich mit dem Mund,
Folg ich Gottes Willen.
Wenn ich Gott erblick'
Überall, in Mutter, Vater,
In allen lieben Menschen,
In Tier und Blume,
In Baum und Stein,
Gibt Furcht mir nichts;
Nur Liebe zu allem,
Was um mich ist.

Children's prayer

From my head to my feet
I am the image of God,
From my heart to my hands
His own breath do I feel;
When I speak with my mouth,
I shall follow God's will
When I see and know God
In my father and mother,
And all good people,
In the animals and flowers,
In trees and stones
Then no harm shall come near me,
Only love shall surround me.

Rudolf Steiner (see p. 26 for exercise using this poem)

Wir reiten geschwinde durch Feld und Wald,
Wir reiten bergab und bergauf.
Und fällt wer vom Pferde, so fällt er gelinde,
Und klettert behend wieder rauf.
Es gcht über Stock und Stein,
Wir geben dem Rosse die Zügel,
Und reiten im Sonnenschein,
So schnell, aus hätten wir Flügel.
Heissa, hurra! Über Stock und über Stein
Und in den Stall hinein.

Traditional (see p. 31 for exercise using this poem)

195

Fein Rösslein,
Ich beschlage dich,
Sei frisch und fromm,
Und wieder komm!
Trag deinen Herrn
Stets treu dem Stern,
Der seiner Bahn
Hell glänzt voran. ...

F. Rückert (see p. 37 for exercise using this poem)

Abendglockengebet

Das Schöne bewundern,
Das Wahre behüten,
Das Edle verehren,
Das Gute beschließen:
Es führet den Menschen
Im Leben zu Zielen,
Im Handeln zum Rechten,

Im Fühlen zum Frieden,
Im Denken zum Lichte;
und lehrt ihn vertrauen
auf göttliches Walten
in allem was ist:
im Weltenall,
Im Seelengrund.

Rudolf Steiner (see p. 44, 183 for exercise using this verse)

Alliteration

Kein Nickel lasse!
An angegebenes sieh innig hin!
Weige Wagnis wenig wegen Wogen Windes!
Bete bittend und tue die Tat!
Gib biegend die Gabe ab.
Kein Nickel lasse sieh, auch im Kasten kleben.
Wenn Wüste Wasser   stauen; wenig wohl wird winzig.
Errette redend den netten Retter redender Erdenrede.

(See p. 69 for excercise using this poem)

Standhaft stell' ich mich ins Dasein
Sicher schreite ich die Lebensbahn
Liebe hege ich in Wesenkern
Hoffnung präge ich in all mein Tun.
Vertrauen lege ich in mein Denken
Diese Fünf führen mich ans Ziel,
Diese Fünf geben mir das Dasein.

Rudolf Steiner (see p. 48 for excercise using this verse)

Aus dem tiefen Erdengrund
Wachs ich hinauf zum
Himmelsrund.

"Aus der Kraft der
Wächst der Baum dem Lichte zu,

Feuer schafft in dem Blut
Rechtest Du mit Mut,

Ohne Rast ohne Ruh
Geht's dem Ziele zu

Die dunkle Tanne wuchs in Ruh
WurzelGar still und Ernst den Sternen zu."

H. Diestel (see p. 62 for excercise using this poem)

Diamanten

Morgenhell auf Gräserspitzen
Kleine Tauesperlen sitzen,
Die da funkeln, die da blitzen,
und Demantenglanz versprühn.

Diese Grashalm-Diamanten
Freun sich stolzerer Verwandten,
Die mit feingeschliffnen Kanten,
In der Königskrone glühn.
...

R. Hamerling (see p. 66 for excercise using this poem)

Die Sonn' erregt das All,
Macht alle Sterne tanzen,
Wirst du nicht auch bewegt,
Gehörst du nicht zum Ganzen.

A. Silesius (see p. 84 for exercise using this poem)

from **Vermächtnis**

Ich liebe die Flamme,
Das Glanzelement,
Im Wetterleuchten,
Im Sterngeflimmer.

Ich liebe den Äther,
Den göttlich-freien,
Wo die Winde, die Wolken,
Die Adler wandern.

Ich liebe die Welle,
Die rauschende,
Sehnsüchtig wallende,
Von Land zu Land.

Ich liebe die Erde,
Das heil'ge Grün,
Wo's hold zu wandeln,
Und noch süsser zu ruhn ist.

...

Geist soll lodern,
Seele sich denen,
Des Herzens Woge soll weiter
   rauschen und klingen
Der Leib soll ruhn.

R. Hamerling (see p. 85 for exercise using this poem)

Der Wolkendurchleuchter:
Er durchleute,
Er durchsonne,
Er durchglühe,
Er durchwärme
   Auch uns.

Rudolf Steiner (See pp. 90, 110 for exercises using this verse)

Du Störenfried lass mich in Ruh,
Hab ich nicht Mut und Kraft wie du.
Ich lach' dich aus und lauf nach Haus
Und ruh' mich bei mir selber aus.

(see p. 99 for English translation)

from **Der Strom**

Tief in waldgrüner Nacht
Ist ein Bächlein erwacht
Kommt von Halde zu Halde gesprungen,
Und die Blumen, sie steh'n
Ganz verwundert und seh'n
In die Augen dem lustigen Jungen. ...

R. Reinick (see p. 129 for exercise using this poem)

from **Lied der Krieger**

War Song

Der Ruf des Herrn,
des Vaters tönt;
Wir folgen gern,
wir sind's gewöhnt.
Geboren sind wir all zum Streit,
Wie Schall und Wind zum Weg bereit.

The call of God,
our father's sound;
We follow, yes!
We're glory bound.
We all are born to fight, to cheer,
Like sweeping wind the path is clear.

J. W. Goethe (see p. 153 for exercise with this poem)

Ecce Homo

In dem Herzen webet Fühlen,
In dem Haupte leuchtet Denken,
 In den Gliedern kraftet Wollen.
Webendes Leuchten,
Kraftendes Weben,
Leuchtendes Kraften:
Das ist der Mensch.

In the heart weaving feeling,
In the head, light of thinking,
In the limbs, strength of will.
Weaving radiance,
 Strength of weaving,
Light of strength: Lo,
This is man.

Rudolf Steiner (see p. 160 for excercise using this verse)

Nachts am Berge
Tanzen Zwerge,
Rasch im Nu!
Tanzen schnelle,
Lachen helle –
Halten Ruh!

H. Diestel (see p. 162 for exercise with this poem)

Wer berät langen Rat,
Kommt zu spät mit der Tat.
Wer geschwind sich besinnt
Und beginnt – der gewinnt!

F. Rückert (see p. 163 for exercise with this verse11)

Ich sah, ich sah, wie die Sonne kam,
Die Erde ganz in die Arme nahm,
In Menschenaugen, in Blütenschalen
Sah ich die Sonne widerstrahlen.

H. Diestel (see p. 172 for exercise with this poem)

Im Atemholen sind zweierlei Gnaden:
Die Luft einziehn, sich ihrer entladen;
Jenes bedrängt, dieses erfrischt;
So wunderbar ist das Leben gemischt.
Du danke Gott, wenn er dich presst,
Und danke ihm, wenn er dich wieder entlässt.

J. W. Goethe (see p. 182 for exercise with this poem)

Thank You

Many thanks to the following people without who's help and encouragement this book could not have appeared:

Christine Allsop, Dr. Andreas Bindler, Ursula Browning, Dylan Galloway, Toby Hawkins, Andrew Henderson, Johanna Kartje, Johannes Kartje, Alberto Llorca, Christian Peter, Trevor Smith, Gordon Walmsley, Alexander Winter (cover painting and design) and Geraldine Winter.

Biographies

Ilse Rolofs
(1903–1981)

Her whole being radiated goodness, especially her lovely calm eyes which bore witness to her great loving heart. She stood before children, patients and therapeutic eurythmy students with the strong will of a healer. She always gave well-prepared lessons on the basis of a clear methodology and her own lively character. All that Ilse Rolofs gave to her colleagues and students out of the creative sources of therapeutic eurythmy enlivened within each of them the enthusiasm for the healing ability of the sounds, forms and rhythms.

Ilse Rolofs had met Rudolf Steiner for the first time at the age of five in her father's house in Thüringen, Germany. Sitting on his lap, she and her brother received the evening prayer for children: "From my head to my hands I am in God's image ..." Shortly after her third birthday, she nearly froze to death which resulted in a long-term apathy. Due to this, she received a "very powerful therapeutic eurythmy finger exercise" which was to help her to incarnate more strongly. This was her first connection to therapeutic eurythmy which only years later would actually be developed.

"The finger exercise was such that I had to pull in each finger strongly one after the other until all five were folded in. In this position I then had to push my hand up and down vigorously from the wrist five times, first the right then the left, then the same process with both hands at the same time: first always each finger separately, beginning with the thumb then with the whole hand."

When her father asked about what profession she should pursue, Rudolf Steiner said that she should, "simply study eurythmy." Obedient, although somewhat reluctant, she went to the only existing eurythmy training in Stuttgart at the age of 16. This was being run by Lory Maier-Smits. After four weeks she was enthusiastic and remained so for the rest of her life. At the age of 18, barely finished with this training, she started teaching eurythmy in a newly founded Waldorf school in Hamburg, Germany, on the advice of Rudolf Steiner. Shortly thereafter, she was called to Stuttgart to learn therapeutic eurythmy from Elisabeth Maier, who died shortly afterwards. She had been bed-ridden at the Dr. Palmer clinic, so Ilse Rolofs practised by her sickbed. She followed her teacher's explanations and corrections until the therapeutic eurythmy exercises "settled" within her. It was a real inner working that bonded the two of them, and Ilse felt Elisabeth Maier to be constantly guiding her work. Her meeting with Trude Thetter in about 1969 enabled her to give of her rich experiences in the therapeutic eurythmy courses held at the Goetheanum in Dornach. This deep friendship joined the two teachers (who were both greatly loved by their students) and helped them to give courses in therapeutic eurythmy over the next seven years from 1969 until 1975. (from: *Mitteilungen aus der Anthroposophischen Arbeit in Deutschland*, 1982 und *Aus der Entstehungszeit der Heileurythmie* Heft 2, Schriftenreihe der Arbeitsgruppe Heileurythmie der Arbeitsgemeinschaft Anthroposophischer Ärzte, 1972)

Trude Thetter

(1907–1982)

Trude Thetter contributed very much to the development of eurythmy and of therapeutic eurythmy. Many students came to her training to receive a strong and solid foothold in the basic elements of artistic and therapeutic eurythmy in order to become properly equipped to carry out their personal eurythmic life goals. Many of these students have become leading personalities in the field of therapeutic eurythmy today.

She was born into an artistic and pedagogically oriented family; her father was a painter. Her uncle, Rudolf Thetter, a well-known magnetopath in Germany, played an important part in her life. At the age of 15 she was introduced to Rudolf Steiner. Two years later Trude was sent to the Waldorf School in Stuttgart with her cousin where she became acquainted with eurythmy.

In 1927 she and Ilona Baltz were given the task by Marie Steiner to found the eurythmy school in Vienna. In 1934 Trude Thetter received her therapeutic eurythmy diploma from Elisabeth Baumann. In 1935, she and Gritli Eckinger founded the Vienna Eurythmy School. Friedl Meangya later joined them.

In 1952 Trude Thetter was asked if she could found a therapeutic eurythmy training in Dornach. She decided to give a six-week course once a year there to fulfil this task. This initiated 21 years of intensive collaboration among many doctors and eurythmists. After these 21 years she held further courses for therapeutic eurythmy in Vienna. In her way of working, Trude Thetter clearly separated the artistic from the hygienic-therapeutic. Through her deep connection to the therapeutic eurythmy she obtained a sense of certainty in her being, and a clear sense for the therapeutic and/or artistic capacities lying dormant within her students. (From: Bodo v. Plato: Anthroposophie im 20. Jahrhundert, Verlag am Goetheanum, Dornach.)

Anne-Maidlin Vogel

(1940–1999)

Anne-Maidlin, one of ten children, was born in Jena, East Germany, and was proud of the town where, she would remind us, Goethe, Schiller, Haeckel and other great Germans worked. Her father was a landscape architect and the only capitalist allowed to own his own land in his town under the Communist regime. At her birth, her father could hold her entire body in the palm of his hand, although she was not premature. He invented the name "Maidlin," meaning "little maiden," and he had predicted months earlier her exact date and hour of birth. She was also proud to tell all who asked that she was born at 11 minutes after 11 o'clock in the morning on the 11th day of the 11th month!

Anne-Maidlin loved life: day-long walks with her husband, food, clothes, her teachers, and of course, her students and patients. She loved and trusted all people. Later in life, this trust in people and her frequent disillusionment wounded her deeply.

As a teenager, she loved to dance and had many dancing partners. For a short time she did some acting as an "extra" in the local theatre group, but this was stopped by her mother when her grades at school dropped dramatically. When she graduated from class 12, she studied weaving for a year and produced some beautifully woven scarves, blankets and dresses.

When she was 21 years old, she and a girlfriend went to a Christian Community weekend conference in the western part of Berlin. On the night before she was to return to Jena, the Berlin Wall was constructed in secret. It was only three feet high at first, separating East from West Berlin. Anne-Maidlin did not return to Jena but stayed in the West and in 1962 began her eurythmy studies with Else Klink at the Stuttgart Eurythmy School.

Norman Francis Vogel joined this school and stage group for a time as pianist, taking a break from his eurythmy studies in Dornach. He met Anne-Maidlin while playing for her eurythmy class. They continued eurythmy studies together and graduated from the Vienna School of Eurythmy in 1965. Anne-Maidlin always had to work during her studies in Vienna, and although often exhausted in school time, she insisted on doing a thorough job in every detail at school and also as a janitor, cleaning the three-story building that included the very primitive apartment that she was allowed in exchange for doing the janitor's job. She was a perfectionist in everything, not least eurythmy.

After a postgraduate year in Vienna, Anne-Maidlin and Norman Francis were invited to join the Zuccoli stage group in Dornach. During this time they both received their therapeutic eurythmy diplomas. It was possible to take part in stage work and still be able to work as therapeutic eurythmists twice a week in nearby homes, and this they did.

Anne-Maidlin married Norman Francis on June 2, 1974. Together they went to Spring Valley, New York, to teach in the eurythmy school, which was then entering its third year.

There they taught for five years, returning to Europe in 1979. In 1981 they began their main life's initiative together, establishing the School of Eurythmy in Stourbridge, England. Francis Edmunds, their good friend and founder of Emerson College was their spiritual mentor. He gave the initial talk that opened the school and came each year to teach a block of lessons to their students until his death in 1989. The school thrived for 17 years, closing in 1998.

During the 17 years in Stourbridge, Anne-Maidlin took on many tasks and became the much-loved therapeutic eurythmist for the children at Elmfield Rudolf Steiner School in Stourbridge as well as for many adult patients. She also taught the students in the Eurythmy School and brought many innovative ideas to them. She became one of the leaders of the Therapeutic Eurythmy Training at Peredur, teaching over 450 students in the 14 years of her work there. Her devotion to eurythmy, her light and warmth-filled enthusiasm, joy and interest in helping each individual she met, her clear step-by-step development of the elements of eurythmy in each class she taught, and her important contributions in the meetings and conferences with other therapeutic eurythmists in the wider area were a source of inspiration for all!

She left behind hundreds of students and many co-workers who will never forget how much they were carried and helped by her constant encouragement in all situations and how health, harmony and joy streamed out from her entire being. She was always serving the Being of eurythmy. She also left behind a husband who can truthfully say that no one could have hoped for or asked for a truer, more devoted wife, co-worker and friend.

About the Coming Generation

About the Coming Generation

"The approaching younger generations come from quite different cosmic worlds than we do. This will increase over time. They bring with them a very strong capacity for thinking, a virtuosity in thinking. This is the greatest temptation and at the same time the greatest ahrimanic attack against Anthroposophy. The danger will be that through an incredible ease of understanding anthroposophical ideas, Anthroposophy itself will get stuck in thinking. Thus an incredible comfort in anthroposophical thinking will develop, but one will not be able to break through to a path of inner development. The only thing that the youth will receive, that will strengthen them in order to withstand this future situation is that they meet up with Anthroposophy on their path of inner development. The path of self-development is the foundation through which study can be guided to reach a true goal. If Anthroposophy is taught as a mere science, it will be harmful. Anthroposophy may never be simply theory; it has to become instantaneous life. If it is allowed to be simply empty teachings, then one kills it and gives it over to Ahriman, the Lord of Death. Today it is much more comfortable for people to think and to adopt a few anthroposophical ideas for oneself than it is to give up one solitary habit. Much more important than all such theoretical knowledge of the content of spiritual science is what happens within our souls, what our souls become through Anthroposophy."

(Oral statements of Rudolf Steiner made to Sybell Petersen and related by Adelheid Petersen in a lecture August, 1950)

"You Too, Uncle Lou"

Anne-Maidlin Vogel and Norman Francis Vogel

Episodes from Their Life Together

Did I see right? It was crazy! I could hardly believe my eyes! She was the only one in the group who always walked on her toes, always turned in the direction she moved in (right, left, forward or backward) – so that she was always walking forward. ALL the others in her class kept facing front and walked sideways to the right or left, backward when walking backward – and her voice – two octaves too high and squeaky! She was already in the second year of the four-year eurythmy training! Boy! – She was far from being "incarnated." She just sort of floated two feet over the earth – always smiling – loving everything and everybody in a childlike manner. This of course was nice – this trusting innocence unfortunately became the source of much pain many years later. This floating about was uncomfortable for me to see. (I played piano for this class for a short time). So I thought to myself – I want nothing to do with this woman.

When she first noticed me, she was also shocked for quite different reasons. She would tell everyone how she saw me each day in the breaks, leaning on my ancient, wooden dash boarded, convertible Mercedes, cigarette dangling from my lips, in my disgusting nylon pullover, vomiting an ugly red color, surrounded by girls – an air of conceit around me. Such a sight for her was most deplorable – she wanted nothing to do with such a person!!!!

These were the first impressions we had of each other. This first inauspicious meeting blossomed into thirty-five years of joyful working, playing and suffering together. I cannot speak for her – she can no longer speak for herself – but I can say one would seldom find today such a co-worker, friend and wife. In those early months of our relationship, when we accidentally crossed each other's path, she would greet me with, "hello, there doctor professor teacher director musician" and bow down in mock reverence. She knew about all my degrees and simply made fun of them (though I knew she was somehow a bit impressed as well).

Recently, a friend of hers in her class at that time told me of the day she invited them all to lunch. Everyone came at the appointed time, but no Maidlin! They waited ten to fifteen minutes. Then in the distance they saw her running towards them, with a load of corn, beans and other vegetables in her arms. A farmer was running close behind, slowly catching up to her before she reached her classmates and her home. The farmer, very angry, stopped her and it looked, from the distance, as if he demanded the return of everything that she had taken from his garden. A long discussion ensued, with much gesticulation of arms coming from Maidlin – (no one could hear what they were saying).

After a time the farmer quietly left and Maidlin continued on to her classmates, and lunch was prepared. In a few minutes the farmer returned, bringing bags full of vegetables to the "poor students who had to work while studying full time." Maidlin had certainly exaggerated in painting a picture of such a painful life situation for the students, to the farmer. The farmer, gave what he gave, with great joy and left feeling he had done a good deed!!

A few months later, the eurythmist, Friedhelm Gillert, was invited to participate in a performance with Ilse Klink and the Stuttgart Ensemble (where Maidlin studied and I played piano). I was very impressed with this eurythmist's way of working, and when he returned home to Italy I followed shortly afterwards, to continue my eurythmy studies with him in his small eurythmy school. (I had begun my studies a year before in Dornach and interrupted them to play for the Klink School of Eurythmy because I needed money to send to my first wife and children who were then in Germany.) However I had to start again from the beginning. Maidlin appeared a month later and joined the 2nd year group.

Very beautiful lessons followed, which we all appreciated. Maidlin lived and helped in the house where Mr. Gillert and his wife lived. This was also the school, with one good-sized room and a smaller room for lessons and practices. I lived in a nearby village, twenty minutes walk to the school. Maidlin and I met in the school at 7:30 every morning before lessons began, and practiced together for over an hour. Next door to the practice room was the kitchen. Mr. and Mrs. Gillert (both eurythmists) would be having breakfast while we practiced.

Even before we practiced, (about 7 a.m.) Maidlin had to take their dog, a giant one, for a walk in a nearby field. Now we decided we would meet in this field each morning, and so we did. She and the dog coming from one end of the field, I from the other end. We were about 150 meters apart. Well, when we caught sight of each other, we dashed to meet with great joy, the dog even happier then we, barking and galloping along. We kept running and running our joy intensifying as we came closer and closer. Then when we were close enough she took a running leap into my arms almost knocking me over. The dog wanted to do the same! The air was filled with laughter and barking and best of all the shining sun streaming out of Maidlin's eyes, which illuminated everything around her even on rainy days. Such joy to be with each other (years later this streaming sun flowing from her eyes would at times turn into streaming tears). After this bubbling euphoric meeting in the field we went on hand in hand to practice together in the eurythmy house.

One day we were called to a meeting. In a very serious mood we were told: "Dr. Steiner found it unproductive to have two people so strongly connected in their astral bodies who were not married to practice eurythmy together with no one else in the room." Poor Maidlin loved her teacher, loved me, and didn't know what to do. Luckily, Lori Meier-Smits, the first eurythmist in the world, was to come to teach us in a week or so. I asked Maidlin to ask her what she thought about it. Had Dr. Steiner made such a comment? I had my doubts. Frau Smits and Maidlin met at the school on the veranda and spoke about many things. I waited in the eurythmy room – I could hear their voices but I was not able to make out what they were saying. Suddenly Frau Smits let out gales of laughter! The meeting ended shortly after this. When I asked Maidlin if she had asked Frau Smits what we wanted to know, Maidlin said: "Yes!" That was when she laughed so hard and long and said, "I never heard Dr. Steiner saying such a thing, and cannot imagine that he ever would have!!" So we continued to practice merrily onward, each morning as before much to the displeasure of our teachers!!!

On weekends we would hitchhike to the many beautiful attractions in this country. We had wonderful experiences at that time. However, our just as wonderful teacher would ask us what we had done on the weekend. We said we were here or there – and enjoyed every minute of it. Then we were asked how we got to those places? "Hitchhiking, of course," we said. We had no car and very little money. "That was a serious mistake. If we wanted to become eurythmists because hitchhiking uses up etheric energy which one needs for eurythmy," we were told. This of course is true – but we had to see these beautiful famous places like Orbino, where Raphael was born, Rome, Assisi, etc., even if it meant sacrificing our etheric bodies. Our dear teacher was not happy with us, and needed each week until Wednesday to overcome his disappointment in our continuing "misbehavior." We learned and improved (perhaps slower, and with less etheric forces) in spite of it all!

This little school had eight or nine students in it. I was the only one in the first year for six months (Anne-Maidlin was in the second year with four others). Then came a second student to my course! How wonderful!. We could do mirror picture forms together. I was no longer alone in the training. She arrived as an angel, a savior, for me.

Maidlin and I worked hard during the week, and had so much joy in going places on the weekends. In everything Maidlin and I were always together. She came from East Germany, with strong connections to Russia. I came from America, with strong feelings for Russia (my grandparents were born in Russia). And so, years later, when we founded the Eurythmy school in England, which was recognized by the Dornach authorities, our students told us how they experienced us as teachers! "Very strong individuals with approaches from so many different sides, but like coming from one soul!" But I'm getting ahead of my story.

After a few months in the eurythmy school in Italy, Maidlin moved in with an Old Italian lady, in a small town just outside of Florence. Señorina Olga was her name – a woman of about 85; small, bony, but full of fire and joy. She was so proud when Maidlin who was tall and beautiful would walk down the village street with her arm in arm, for all to see! In the winter, Olga carried a real small iron coal stove – "stuffina" – heater under her apron to keep herself warm. It actually had burning coal in it! How it never burned her, I don't know! I was always worried that it would set her dress on fire!

Once a week I was invited to visit Anne-Maidlin, at Señorina Olga's apartment for a rather short supper together (all three of us). Afterwards Maidlin and I went to her room and closed the door. We simply just talked quietly together, nothing else. After about half an hour, Señorina Olga shouted out, half-crying, half-laughing, half in despair and very loud, "Basta amore, Señor. Por favor. Basta amore." – In a quivering voice she began to fake loud crying (she was a real actress), "Prego, Señor – basta amore-oi, oi!". We'd burst into laughter and I'd come out and leave. She, Olga, half-crying, half-laughing to herself, asked me to please not do it again.

For a few months a fellow student and I lived together in a small two-storey four-room house near the village where Maidlin lived. It was a twenty minutes walk from the Piazza Michelangelo, which was close to the eurythmy school.

One day this colleague said to me, "I've observed, Herr Vogel (although we knew each other quite well, he never called me by my first name, which bothered me a bit, and made me call him by his first name even louder than normal!) – "That you drink far too much coffee." (I was drinking at least 10-12 cups a day, strong and black, no sugar.) I said, "Yes, perhaps, but I like it and I need it." "Well," said he, "you're so addicted to it, you couldn't stop now anyway which you should, even if you wanted to." I answered rather proudly, "I certainly could stop if I wanted to – but –I don't want to!" At which point he laughed very loud and long. That laughing, I'll never forget. It got right into my veins and arteries, and then I said angrily, " Alright, I will stop – and today!" At which point he laughed still louder and longer – which of course made me determined to stop – a wonderful pedagogical trick he implemented with success. I said to his amazement, "What do we bet?" After he repeated his disbelief in my decision, we bet a candy bar. And – I stopped that day! But the next day I could not get out of bed until almost noon. Fortunately it was a winter holiday time.

It gradually got better, and 4-5 days later Anne-Maidlin and I went on our hitchhiking holiday. After a week, somewhere far from home, I developed a very large infection near my right ear on my head for which I had to take penicillin. To help dissolve the negative effect of it Maidlin gave me juniper berries; first day one berry, second day two berries and so on until seven. Then on the eighth day, six berries, ninth day five berries and so on until back to one berry. Maidlin said to me: "These berries are known to have a blood purifying quality!" She was so careful that on the first day, after taking one berry, she had me sit in the sun for one minute. On the second day when I took two berries I had to sit in the sun for two minutes, etc. Such loving care, such tender hands and fingers touching my head! I felt she must have been sent to the earth as my angel's helper!

After one and a half years in this small school, a fellow student told me I should go to Vienna to finish my training. I belonged there, he said. I never even knew there was a training there, but I went to visit at a pre-arranged time, rang the bell and a woman answered who had cleaning material in her hands, and a cloth tied around her head. I said, "Oh, I'm sorry to interrupt your work. Can you tell me where I can find Fraulein

Thetter, please?" (The school founder and leader.) After a short pause she said with a smile, "I am Fraulein Thetter, and you must be Herr Vogel." I couldn't imagine this woman being the founder and leader of a eurythmy school until I looked into her eyes, which shone like stars, dark brown eyes! So we met. I joined the school: telephoned Maidlin – who was still in the other school, which was soon to move to another country – and said she should come at the end of the term. Well, then the drama began!

My first lesson in the second year class with Fraulein Thetter in tone eurythmy was a catastrophe for me. We clapped and stepped very simple sixteenth- and seventeenth-century music examples – "Ping-Pong Music" we called it, a Maidlin invention – and it seemed to me we did very little else except walking figure eights and very harmonious kidney-shaped forms which Fraulein Thetter had made up. This clapping and stepping really bothered me in the beginning. I could do it after one try. I was a musician, after all. The others in the class needed to repeat it at least 10 to 15 times before they could do it. In other words, I was bored. Added to that was our teacher's attitude. She sat motionless on high chair, wearing sunglasses; (there was no sun in the room), saying nothing except "Once more." Then at the end of the lesson she added: "Practice this thoroughly and we see each other next time" (in two days).

So – so – that was not for me – no – not at all. We had such interesting, exciting music in the small school from where I had come. That evening, I called Maidlin and told her to stay where she was. I was returning and would move with the school at the end of the year!!

Next day our class was to experience Friedl Meangya teaching us speech eurythmy. That was another world; fantastic, exciting. She moved with us, bellowed out the texts we were to learn –- explained so much in such an interesting and deep way. After this lesson I ran to the telephone and told Maidlin she should come after all – the speech eurythmy teacher was great. Next day we had Trude Thetter in the tone eurythmy. Again I was bored. Again I went to the telephone, " No, Maidlin, don't come, it won't work," So back and forth for three weeks, at least. Poor Maidlin didn't know what she should do. Yes – No – Yes – No. (I didn't either) But I stuck it out and slowly realized that it was how one clapped and stepped the music pieces, that was the important thing. It took a deep sensitivity that one could only slowly develop. This and many other intimate things, inch by inch, revealed themselves to me. So, Maidlin finally came, and the next three years in Vienna were the most joyful years of our lives – or certainly of my life!

When we first came to Vienna, we had to get a student card called "Sichtvermerk" from the government at the appropriate building and on the appropriate floor. When we arrived there was a line; a long line. I counted that we were the 44th and 45th persons in line. Well, two hours later, the office closed, leaving about twenty of us to come back the next day. This happened to us again on the second day, but before the office closed (we were then number 28 and 29), a woman entered the corridor, dressed up to the hilt in a long gown, high heels, fur scarves, and all made up. To our amazement – from the end of the line – she klip-klopped with her heels to the front, knocked on the office door, entered and came out three minutes later waving her "Sichtvermerk" in her hand. She was proudly smiling while we were all frowning as we looked with open mouths in disbelief. Anne–Maidlin said, "That's it!" We went home immediately, and returned the next day. Maidlin was all dressed up as if going to a ball. Klip-klopping to the front of the line, she knocked on the door, walked in and came out smiling waving her "Sichtvermerk"!! (I waited and finally got in two hours later.)

Each morning during the week we would arrive at the school at 7:30 a.m. – ring the bell to get into the apartment building, then walk up the three flights to the eurythmy school floor; then ring that bell, which of course woke up the student who lived in the school who would let us in with a sour face. We excused ourselves over and over again. We simply had to practice, practice, and practice before lessons began! After a few weeks of this, and with grand ceremony, the special favour was granted us to have a key of our own! I can't do justice in words to the exhilarated feelings and enthusiasm we had in practicing together for one and half-hours before school started! Oh, yes, we were exhausted by 5:30 or 6:00 p.m., when lessons ended, but with a creative, exhausted feeling – actually refreshing! Then came Friday evening! Each week it came and from that moment on until Monday morning we lived in the world of Viennese culture. And what a world that was, and still is, mostly.

Opera, concerts, theatre – such choices each week – unbelievable and incomparable to any other city Maidlin or I knew about! And the walks in the Viennese woods – yes, Vienna, the workplace of Bruckner, Beethoven, Mozart, Berg, Schoenberg and many others – Vienna, where the women stallholders on the "Nasch-markt" (marketplace) street after street stand after stand sold vegetables, fruits, cheese, fish, meat, exotic herbs to buy, etc. One of these stallholders would ask us if we were going to the opera that night because we should. She would then tell us that in the opera that night so and so was being sung and the famous singer from Prague was singing – the best of the lot, and then the stallholder would sing the one or two main arias from the opera! They knew their operas and singers better than we did! But you were not allowed to help yourself to the fruit you wanted to buy. If you began to do this, as we did at first, you would get your hand slapped and an angry loud voice would say: "Na, na – das mache i" (No, no – I do it!) After the very first time we discovered why. The counter-women always had some half-rotten fruit hidden under the counter. Every five pieces of fruit included one bad one from under the counter. That was why the prices were cheaper than in the stores. So – we accepted it all, with knowing smiles. It was all part of the game! We would set out with our sacks on the twenty-minute walk to the " Nasch-markt." We would look through the streets, picking out this and that. So much choice, another cultural aspect of Vienna. It belonged and still does belong to Viennese life: the joy, the laughter, bubbling through each Saturday morning. We tumbled with it – were carried by it! Such a wonderful life it was for us.

One night, in 1972, during a performance of Tosca the greatest singer of her generation, Galina Vischnevskaya – (we were in the audience) – during a very dramatic scene in which she was fighting off a man who was trying to seduce her, was pushed by him against a table. Her body being bent over backwards, just a little too far over the table caused her hair wig to catch on fire from the lit candles on it! A stagehand came running onto the stage to rip off the burning wig as the curtains quickly closed. And we, the audience, in a state of shock, waited for the announcement that the rest of the performance would be cancelled. But, wonder of wonders! Fifteen minutes later it was announced – not what we expected, that the performance would continue in five minutes! Well, what an uproar of hurrahs when the curtain finally opened: The orchestra and the wrestling of the two performers just took up where it had left off – as if nothing had ever happened – a rare artistic grip! And, of course, as Galina came out onto the stage, such uproar of clapping and bravos – that for two to three minutes one could not hear the orchestra!

Years later, in her book *A Russian Story,* she refers to that experience and says: a week after that night, she suddenly almost broke down – and then realized how it had taken its toll. She first noticed her burnt fingernail ends, and remembered how she tried to put out the fire with her hands…. But at the time she insisted that the show must go on. She was a genuine artist.

Then there was the performance in 1973, of David Oistrach, the outstanding Russian violinist of his generation! He would play two of the unaccompanied suites of Bach for violin. Of course, we were in the audience for this one too. Well, watching him play, leaning back on his heels, so relaxed and easy, he looked like he was playing for a New England Summer Barn Dance. It was difficult for me to reconcile his facile way of playing together with the deeply beautiful cosmic sound coming from his instrument – and such difficult music played in such an almost " who cares" look about him. A real genius and an unforgettable experience! I thought, that is how eurythmy should be performed. The eurythmist should always look relaxed and joyful. (Maidlin would tell students; "It's easy-peasy" when they thought a particular part of the lesson was difficult).

In our last year of the eurythmy training at the end of each morning Frau Meangya would ask who would come in the afternoon for their speech solo (one person each day would volunteer). Fine – We'll begin at 2:00 p.m.! 2:00 p.m.! But it was already after 1:00 pm. and we were all in classes since 9:00 a.m. with one twenty-minute break. (Maidlin and I, of course, since 7:30 a.m.). For Frau Meangya it was no problem. She only needed half an hour to eat her lunch of sandwich and coffee, and then she'd be as fresh as if she had just started the day! We didn't have the strength to start so early in the afternoon. We came of course, half dead and fumbled our way through our solos, half asleep. (Maybe it was better so – very relaxed and sleepy). That generation of teachers had endurance that no one today could match! Oh, there is so much to tell! It is difficult to put into words the mood we were both in.

Of course, how can I forget? The Vienna Balls. My, what an experience each February. They always took place in different "Burgs" in Vienna, either in castles, or in the opera house or in the concert hall – gigantic rooms, large orchestras, even a Dixieland Band in one of the smaller rooms. Women dressed as formally as possible, with long white gloves that virtually went up to their armpits! Men in tuxedos and tails. My, oh my! They started at 9:00 or 10:00 p.m. and ended in the morning at 4:00 or 5:00 a.m.!! Anne-Maidlin taught me how to hold my head still for the waltz, in turning, and just snap it suddenly, every few seconds – so as to not get dizzy. (She loved dancing almost as much as eurythmy.) When I tried the sudden jerk of the head – it's true, I didn't get dizzy going round and round in the same direction – just occasionally sprained my neck. Then at 5:00 a.m. we'd go out into the empty streets, exhausted, happy and HUNGRY! Nothing would open until 7:00 a.m. – it was usually an hour's walk to get home, and we didn't want to go home.

We were really on a high, without alcohol! So we wandered around singing, dancing in the streets, until something opened somewhere. Then eating and finally returning home. We plopped on the bed completely worn out and joyful. We usually went to two balls each season. There were at least six to eight during the month of February, and only during this month. The experience of the Balls were as if we were on another planet. They had nothing to do with anything else we did. It was a world onto itself.

Opera going on weekends was always a drama of momentous proportions! If there was a famous singer imported from Russia or America or elsewhere, four of us at least, would have to get together who wanted to go, and make a plan, if we wanted the first row standing room in the gallery. In this first row only, we could sit on the ledge behind us and still see the whole stage. These places were limited to about a hundred people. (Gallery tickets in 1965 cost ten pence each.)

So, the plan was made – two of us would begin by standing in the line on Saturday at 8:00 a.m. the latest, for the performance that evening. There were always two dozen or more people who had spent the entire night before in line. Then an hour or two later, two others of our group would relieve the first two who had started at 8:00 a.m. – and so on- exchanging every one or two hours. Doors opened at 6:30 p.m. but by 4:00 p.m. the queue was already round the corner, about three hundred to four hundred people strong.

In this long exhausting wait, we became well acquainted with the people in front and behind us. We shared sandwiches, drinks and conversation. Sometimes we learned from each other intimate details of our lives. The Austrians were so friendly and warm hearted. All of us being in the same boat made it conducive to good conversation. When we finally got our unnumbered tickets we had to make a mad dash up four flights of stairs with a herd of people. We raced like animals in order to get those "golden" standing room "seats."

Then in the middle of our stampede we were suddenly stopped short in our tracks! A rope was pulled across at the next landing and acted as a fence, No one knew why we were stopped. It was a deep, dark mystery! This nervous waiting lasted about ten minutes, and then, just as suddenly as we were stopped, the rope was taken away and the race continued.

Some of the friends we made earlier, standing in line, became our adversaries, making large, leap-like lunges, galloping for those precious standing-room "seats." Others became real friends, who, if faster than us, would save space for us in the much sort after standing room "seats."

If we got on to the standing line too late, and the gallery standing was all sold out (where one could sit in the front row and be able to see), we'd have to take the back of the main hall standing room downstairs. Then we would amuse ourselves whilst waiting for the program to begin by sitting on the floor inside the main entrance to the auditorium and watching the feet of those who came by: how they walked; quickly, slowly, bow-legged, Charlie Chaplin-like, limping or whatever. We would then discuss what each needed in curative eurythmy. Then just before the lights went down, we'd stand up and look at all the backs of the heads of people. We would choose one or two and try to imagine the size and shape of their noses according to the shape and size of their heads. Then in the intermission, we'd watch that person as he or she turned to go out – and, lo and behold, sometimes we were quite right! (Sometimes we had differences of opinions and sometimes both of us were very wrong!!) Nevertheless, it kept us practicing observation. This was a wonderful contrast to the extremely long and serious mood of the eurythmy training during the week. In fact, the joyful culture-filled weekends helped us in our eurythmy work. It relaxed us and gave us the contrast needed for our souls and spirits!

I must tell you about an experience we had in one of our speech eurythmy practices! There were ten students in our class, eight women and two men (I being one of them). At the beginning of the session, we were all in a very very serious and religious mood – except for the other man! We nine wanted to practice a very spiritual poem, with a silent Vortakt (introduction), to be done in a circle, facing each other, facing the centre of the circle.

The other man refused to take part, and hid behind the curtain which went halfway up to the ceiling, closing off a part of the room where the chairs which were brought out for the Friday night members' meetings taking place in that same room were stored. So, as I said, he hid behind the curtain and stayed quiet there as we began the silent movements in the circle. Our mood was really beautifully serious and concentrated. Suddenly, from over the top of the curtain flew a banana peel, and landed right in the middle of our holy circle. What a shock! Of course we couldn't continue. He had won. He came out with a sheepish grin on his face, and we practiced a light-hearted joyful poem, just what he had wanted! Some of us holier ones were very angry with him and didn't speak to him for days afterwards – others thought it hilarious!

I remember the singing, the end of term festivals, the Christmas plays, etc. We were one happy family, and our mother was Trude Thetter!

Now Anne-Maidlin lived near me, and was the janitor of the corner apartment house. (For that work, she received a free apartment.) It could hardly be called an "apartment." It was a tube, long and thin, divided by a door. One part was the so-called kitchen, (water was only in the hallway, and only cold water) and the other, the bedroom. Both parts together were about two yards wide and six yards long. There also was no heating, apart from an electric heater, and the toilet was in the hallway. We made our scrumptious meals on a two-burner stove. We ate all our meals together, as I lived in still more primitive accommodations. My "summer house" was a tiny 2 x 4 yards room which stood in the courtyard of a large apartment building. It had no water and no toilet, both of which were in the apartment hallway, and I had to go through the courtyard to get there. But I did have a wood stove, one electric light and a beautiful nut tree just outside my window which I adored. That was it. On winter mornings it was difficult to get the place warmed up early enough to do my "foot writing" exercises. Trying to write a part of Goethe's *Faust* with a pencil between my big toe and the next one at 6:00 a.m. in January in 0° temperature was quite a painful ordeal, especially when I wrote one or two sentences each day in mirror picture with the left foot as well. A shivering, shaking writing was the result. But I gritted my teeth and did it! I looked forward to the warmer weather to come! An hour or so earlier (4:30 a.m.) four horses drawing a long wagon from the milk collection depot which was housed between our two accommodations clip-clopped onto the streets to deliver the barrels of milk to the large supermarkets. Such a beautiful klip-klop-klip-klop; especially on snowy mornings. To hear this reassuring sound with no other sound to be heard was pure magic!

In the graduating year, each of us had to learn the usual required solos. Now came the last three to four months before graduation. I was already sick of my tone solo and needed help badly! I told Trude Thetter I knew all the three pages of Dr. Steiner's forms for the piece (I called this one spaghetti forms as it looked like tangled spaghetti on a plate). I told her in addition that I also knew all the tones, but my arms felt like two sticks – in fact, I felt nothing! "I need your help, Fraulein Thetter, please!" She told me, "In two days I go to Dornach for a month to teach in the curative eurythmy training there. Practice it thoroughly, I'll see you in four weeks. Bye bye." Off she went. Boy, was I angry. "Practice it," she'd said. But how? I had no idea!! I told everyone, "I'm not doing that Beethoven piece, even if it means I don't get a diploma! I cannot hear it any more!"

The next day, the loving pianist, Frau Stemberger, invited me to her apartment that coming Sunday for tea and cakes. Of course I went, how could one refuse Vienna's cakes! After a while she said, "Norman, would you just listen to your piece that I will play for you now?" "No!" I said sharply, "I cannot bear to hear it." Soon I left, thanking her for the tea, cakes and company. The following Sunday, she invited me again, and after a while asked if she could just play the first eight bars. I gave a reluctant okay and noticed how beautifully she played. On the third Sunday, as she played, and got me to move in her small living room saying, "Don't do tones, just listen and move freely." The fourth Sunday I liked the piece almost as much as the cakes, especially because I was doing no tones or forms (what a relief!). When Fraulein Thetter returned she wanted to see the piece. I said, "there is nothing to see – no form, no tones." She looked at it anyway and said afterwards, "Beautiful. Now we can begin to work – you are finally listening!"

At various times in Vienna, when we were both still students, I would come down with asthma attacks, especially when we went on holidays for a few days in the nearby country-side. One of my worst attacks was when we went to a special part of the Austrian country-side that was supposed to help asthmatics, and where there was also a sanatorium for respiratory illnesses. Well, for me, this place had the opposite effect. I had to enter their famous sanatorium and follow a special diet for two or three days until I was well enough to return to Vienna which was a two-hour train ride away. Whenever I had an attack out-side Vienna, it went away within days after returning to the city. Except at one time, when I had the attack in Vienna itself. It was a very bad attack, and I had to leave the school for three weeks. I took the inhaler for the first time in my life. It relieved my breathing in the beginning for two to three hours. After three days for one to two hours, and five days later, I was inhaling every five minutes! Then I said "Whoa, wait a minute – this cannot go on or I will suffocate in one more hour" and so I stopped using it. I had to sit, completely still, bend over forward, not moving a muscle for hours until it very slowly let up. Maidlin would take me for very slow short walks during this time. Of course the ice-making machine next door to where I lived, which had a common wall with one of my walls, didn't help matters, going on with a rumbling racket from 3:00 to 5:00 a.m., twice a week, making my wall slowly drip with water.

And my dearest Anne-Maidlin? What did she experience? How did she react to my asthma attacks? Always the same. She stood by me like a loving mother – concerned, pro-tective; always finding new ways to help. For example, with my bronchial asthma, she had read somewhere that the patient should be "whipped" for five to six minutes on the bare back with stinging nettle leaves – young, fresh leaves because they're stronger. She did this for me, which was very painful and caused swelling, redness and itching for hours after-ward. But it did get things moving in my bronchial tubes! This treatment often helped me for days as also the various teas that she made from leaves, and not from tea bags. She would insist on the freshly picked leaves when possible. When not available, she'd buy dried leaves in a pharmacy. She was a real friend – my only real friend who was devoted to me – and I thank her every day for the thirty-five years we had together.

When we were still in Vienna, I would go two or three times a year to America to visit my children and my first wife. I usually went for two weeks. When I returned, I'd find Anne-Maidlin slightly ill, but as happy to see me as I was to see her. Yes, she missed me as much as I missed her when she or I went away. This loneliness when we were apart from each other, even for short intervals of time, was always there throughout all the years we were together.

Vienna was a dream world. Did it really happen? Were we really there? Or did we dream it all? It sometimes seems we dreamed it. How thankful we were to experience it. Toward the end of our first stay there (1964-1966), I once asked Trude Thetter if she could show me or tell me how I could come deeper into the Tone A. (Why A, I no longer know). She answered, "Yes." Then followed a short pause. I became filled with expectant joy. Then, she led me to the nearest wall in the eurythmy room (I still remember today exactly what wall and what spot. I saw it again a year or so ago). She stood me up against it with my back to it, put my arms in the A angle over my head and said, "That, dear Norman, is the deep significance of the Tone A – practice it thoroughly!" (She always said, "Practice it thoroughly"). Then she left the room and left me with my arms hanging in the air – my soul so disillusioned – disappointed I knew all that! Every eurythmist knows all that! What a shallow answer – she just doesn't know, I thought. I left the room mumbling a "thank you" between my teeth, utterly crestfallen. (Years later, I woke up to the fact that the outwardly simplest movements given by Rudolf Steiner can lead to deep insights if really practiced with strong consciousness and concentration!) So, now I sincerely thank you, Trude Thetter.

At the end of our training in Vienna, we stayed an extra year for artistic work. At the same time we were able to finish our curative eurythmy training with Trude Thetter – with just an additional three month course in Dornach with other teachers. Leaving Vienna was very hard for us both. When we afterwards hitchhiked in holiday time and saw a car with a "W" beginning its license number we would wave to the driver as he went by and clap and laugh because we new that car came from Vienna. "Look Maid, there is a W on his license – Vienna (Wien) – hooray!" And we jumped up and down.

After this extra year in Vienna, we were invited to be part of the Zucolli Stage Group in Dornach in Switzerland. So we reluctantly left, looking forward to new experiences. However, before we left, we made it clear to Trude and Friedl that if there was a chance that we could be helpful in Vienna, we would be very interested in returning! Both Trude and Friedl seemed happy to hear this from us. We arrived in Dornach, found suitable quarters, took part in performances and finished our Curative Eurythmy training. We were able to practice Curative Eurythmy in two separate homes for the handicapped about an hour's distance from Dornach.

Fortunately we could also take part in graduate studies taught by many of the famous great artists of that time, mostly pupils of Rudolf Steiner. These were personalities such as Frau Zucolli, Lea Van der Pals, Friedl Simmons-Thomas, Marie Savitch, Ilone Schubert and many others. However, it was no longer the wonderful family feeling as in Vienna. Oh, no. We all had to fend for ourselves. But, we did manage to have a group of five of us who worked independently of the official stage group, and were able to get a program together to bring to four or five homes nearby. That was good work for us. We learned a lot. No one except ourselves to tell us what and how to do it! In this way we probably learned more than we did in the big, famous Zucolli Stage Group.

At the end of the year, the three leading eurythmy personalities from Vienna - Trude Thetter, Friedl Meangya and Liesl Gergerly – came to Dornach to talk to us about working in Vienna. Anne-Maidlin was offered a full time job as a eurythmy teacher in the Mauer Waldorf School. I was offered to teach public classes, and later, to help in the eurythmy school. I said, after much thinking about it, that I just couldn't do it now, much to my regret and apparently theirs. I had to stay longer in Dornach and then go on to Emerson College, where I had been offered a eurythmy teaching job. Of course, the three from Vienna were shocked at my decision and directly thought that Anne-Maidlin would follow me to England. She asked for a day to think about it, and went immediately by herself to Dr. Steiner's Representation of Man statue (the Christ statue) in the Goetheanum. The next day we met again and – lo and behold – Maidlin said she would come to Vienna. Again a shock. No one (least of all myself) had ever dreamed that she would separate herself from me. I was sad. They were happy. And thus began our three year separation from each other, except for holidays when we always met. I found a letter I wrote to her during this time which ended "I always did love you, I love you now and always will love you! You are the love of my lives!" Anne-Maidlin's three years without me in Vienna, teaching the class eurythmy and curative eurythmy with individual children was probably the happiest working time of her life! In the years we were together before this three year "separation," she sometimes felt a little "afraid" of me – or, better as she said, she couldn't find a certain amount of independence from me. Now these three years gave her a security, a certain self-knowledge, a doing without wondering if Norman would approve. Dr. Gergerly, one of the leading personalities of that Waldorf School and a good friend of Anne-Maidlin's, told me years later that the five years she taught in the school were the high point of the eurythmy teaching there.

On one of our holidays, I visited her in Vienna – after not seeing her for six to eight months. It must have been her third year of teaching there. I noticed something in her, around her, that was not visible on our earlier meetings. Another shock, for me at least. She met me at the train – and what did I see? A woman dressed in black, with high black boots, clicking her heels on the ground as she took big, slow steps towards me, to greet me, warmly but with a proudly held head – altogether looking like a beautiful, well-trained horse. The natural uprightness she always had, but this "holier than thou" look about her gave me a fright, and I said, rather excitedly, "Maidlin, where are you? What are you doing?" She didn't understand at first, so I proceeded to explain how she was a bit caught in the trap of hierarchical divisions, which could happen so easily (even amongst Anthroposophists) and especially in old-fashioned Vienna. Sure, she was loved in the school by everyone – she was love incarnated – but in this case, it went a bit to her head.

Still, I was so happy that she was so happy. After the three years, during which time I was a member of Marguerite Lundgren's London Stage Group, taught besides in Emerson College, and in the Wynstones and Michael Hall Waldorf Schools, I decided to return to

Vienna. There we remained for two more years. I taught curative eurythmy part-time in the same school as Maidlin, and we both took part in the stage work directed by Trude Thetter and Friedl Meangya.

I want to tell you about two experiences I had whilst teaching in Wynstones and in Michael Hall while I was in England, during our separation. The first year, the work at Wynstones went well. I had 10 volunteers from Class Nine who wanted extra lessons (besides the normal lessons). They arrived twice a week before school began, each morning, all boys, zooming up to the eurythmy room entrance on their motorbikes, dressed in black leather jackets and trousers – changing into eurythmy shoes. With jackets and trousers kept on, they were ready in a circle to begin at 7:45 in the morning; very early for the English! In one lesson, I went very deeply into just one sound for the entire thirty minutes, and afterwards I thought to myself. "Next time, if they come again, I must have much more variety. It must have been boring for them, although they were good about it." Well, next time came and before we began, they asked me please to repeat what we had done the last time, so that they could get it better. Wow, what a wonderful surprise! So we did. They were happy. I was happy. And the whole world looked brighter for me for that entire week!

Michael Hall was another story! I had to teach Class Eleven. Those "children," in general, came from wealthier parents. They were more like city children, being close to London – and consequently knew everything. The Wynstones pupils had nature behind them, in them, around them, and were more open to others, to the world of surprises, etc. The Michael Hall pupils were simply more easily dissatisfied with what was offered to them, and eurythmy lessons were not their favorite subject. After three or four weeks, I decided to divide the class in two: those who really wanted to do eurythmy with me (seven of them) and, with the others (nine of them), we would recite a poem together once a week. So it began – one lesson a week of eurythmy for the seven; once a week speaking a long, dramatic poem for the other nine. This went well for about a month. The group doing the poem got more and more excited and interested. One of them brought a small tom-tom to occasionally use in building up to dramatic moments. Then a pause, and someone else in the group played a few notes on a trumpet. It was really becoming something – so much so that when the seven who were doing the eurythmy got wind of it, they wanted to join in as well, and stop the eurythmy. So that was that. I had the entire class reciting the poem in different groups, in different ways, and we presented it to the upper school children one afternoon. That was my "eurythmy" experience at the Michael Hall Waldorf School!

I returned to Vienna in 1971. Once again we experienced the Vienna Balls, the Nascht-Markt, going to the opera, to concerts and to the theatre just as it was when we were students. My daughter came from America for a three month visit. She studied the piano with a well–known teacher in Vienna. We had some good times together. Then she returned to America. At the end of two years in Vienna, on the Whitsunday weekend, we were married.

Adam Bittleston, the Christian Community priest in Forest Row, happened to be in Stuttgart at the time, and he was able to come to Vienna to marry us in 1974.

Twenty minutes before the ceremony was to begin, I became very nervous and unsure and spoke to Adam about it. I told him I couldn't go through with it. After all, I was already more or less a failure as a husband and as a father. I had walked out on my first wife and my children who were then eight and ten years old. I loved my children very much, and often cried for them, but I simply couldn't return. I told Adam all this and said, "I'm just not suited to being married, to being a husband." "Well," he answered," I must go through with it now. You'll have many years to learn how to be a husband." So after much persuasion, I did go through with it. (I did love Anne-Maidlin very much, and that's why I wanted to spare her the agony of being married to someone like me!) Because of my doubts and talk with Adam, the ceremony was twenty minutes late in starting.

The wedding was a joyous affair. Maidlin's children from the Waldorf School sang some songs for her, but the ceremony itself was in English. Poor Anne-Maidlin couldn't understand a word of it! I had to poke her at the appropriate time to stand, sit and say, "I will," etc. At the reception afterwards, there were so many people! She was loved by everyone. She loved everyone. Out of this mood of love and trust born out of her innocence, through which she believed everyone, she gradually awakened through painful experiences. Yet she was able to keep a happy enthusiasm for her patients, co-workers, friends, and even tried her best to cover up the pain and disappointments that came to her, from others and myself.

So in 1974 we were married, and were invited to teach in the two-year-old Eurythmy School in Spring Valley, New York! But, Anne-Maidlin needed the "green card" to be able to even enter America! Oh, what a drama! Because she was from East Germany, she was suspected of being a Communist, and she was not allowed to come with me! So when I arrived in America without her, I called the appropriate office in Washington D.C. and screamed on the telephone to some secretary, "But she's my wife," I was told, "Yes we know, but they just have to check her out. It'll be just a few more days," The few days stretched into two weeks, and I called again and said I wanted to speak to the one in charge of all of this business. He wasn't in, of course, and then I said: "If she is not allowed in, in the next three days, I will go to the newspapers and speak to my lawyer." Two days later, her "green card" came through.

We spent each summer doing replacement curative eurythmy, in many clinics in Germany. At that time (1974-1979) it paid very well. We learned and learned and learned, and became refreshingly exhausted by the time the new school year began in September.

After a mix-up with living accommodations, we were given half of a large house on top of one of the main hills in the Anthroposophical settlement, which was three miles south of the rather ugly town of Spring Valley. On the adjoining hill was (and is) the Anthroposophical old people's home. There were two people who were particularly important for us. One was the wife of a well-known Anthroposophical composer in Dr. Steiner's time –

Egon Lustgarten – who had died many years earlier. She cooked lunches for us two times a week. That helped greatly for our work was varied and continuous all day. Also, Anne-Maidlin had to learn English, which took much of her strength. Frau Lustgarten was lively and cheery, and was filled with stories of the good old days. It was supportive, especially for Anne-Maidlin, because we always spoke German when she was with us during those lunches. The other old person was Gladys Hahn – a very lively retired curative eurythmist. We three would meet where the two hills joined (the one where we lived, the other where the old people's home was), to discuss difficulties in the community; the world situation; how one should or could meditate better, or whatever seemed important at the time. We would slowly approach each other from a distance. From the sides of the two hills we saw each other coming closer, closer – she from one side, we from the other; it felt like the beginning of a world conference, between two mighty nations, two mighty leaders! We had a good laugh over the idea!

Now Gladys came to the Fellowship Community thinking she was going to die in a few months – so she gave almost everything away that she owned. She arrived with two knives, two forks, two spoons, two pairs of underwear, two dresses, two coats, two pairs of stockings, two pairs of shoes, two blouses, (Noah's Ark), perhaps ten books – and no more. Well, she died ten years later (about 90 years old), but she was proud not to have brought anything else and kept to just the things she had originally taken with her. She said she was happy with so few things because she didn't have to waste time trying to decide what to wear or use.

Then there was the occasion when we invited all the students for coffee and cake, for Anne-Maidlin's birthday. A week before we told them the date and the time. Oh, Anne-Maidlin went to so much trouble to make it very special; homemade cakes, each napkin folded like a flower. We put two tables together for the twenty students we had at the time. The invitation was for 4:00 p.m. Well, 4:00 p.m. came and went, 4:30, 5:00 p.m., and no one appeared over the horizon. Anne-Maidlin began to cry as we slowly and sadly cleared up. What had happened? We couldn't imagine. That evening and the next morning, I went personally to see the students (it was Sunday). They had all forgotten!! They were so embarrassed and sad. (We should have reminded them, as we had told them a whole week ahead.) So the next day they all came, unannounced, bringing armfuls of flowers, presents, food, singing, etc. What an impression that made on Anne-Maidlin. Oh, how happy she was! All was forgiven. It fostered a strong connection between her and the students.

New York is 30 miles from Spring Valley, so we, of course, took advantage of the Friday and Saturday nights of the opera and the concerts in the city. First, supper with my mother and her devoted second husband in their apartment on W18th Street. Then, before leaving we would say goodbye over and over again, with my mother and stepfather waving to us and screaming out their farewell from their 2nd floor window as we would drive off to Lincoln Center. Such culture again! The programs were of the same high quality as in Vienna, but the mood was not. In Vienna the air was filled with art and culture. It was much stronger than in New York, with its matter-of-fact audience. Yes, I do believe it was the audience in Vienna that created the heart warmth and joy. Though the New Yorkers couldn't quite match it, still, the performances were quite wonderful! I am terribly thankful for it all!

We left Spring Valley after five years, (Maidlin did not like America) and were guests for three months in the new Curative Eurythmy Training in Stuttgart, a very rewarding time. We, though especially Anne-Maidlin, had a lot of joy and enthusiasm to learn, to discover. Then in September 1981 we were invited to Stourbridge, England, where we began our major work together; seventeen years building up, from almost nothing, a eurythmy school that was recognized by the Section for Music, Eurythmy and Art in Dornach, Switzerland – the centre of the Anthroposophical movement founded by Rudolf Steiner. But, at first, we wanted to have the school in connection with the Canterbury Waldorf school. It was always very important for us that eurythmy students had in their first two years of training biodynamic gardening as part of the weeks' program. (Twice a week for one and a half hours each time.) Since there was, and still is, a fabulous farm near that Waldorf school, we thought there would be a perfect opportunity! However, after meeting with the teachers and the farmer, it was thought impractical – because the gardens needed much attention and work just in the summer, when the students were away – to earn money in their home country or elsewhere. (Almost never was it possible to earn enough in England). So we reluctantly said goodbye. Through a eurythmy couple who were my students at Emerson College years earlier, who were working in the Stourbridge area, we were persuaded to move and begin the Eurythmy Training at Elmfield Waldorf School in Stourbridge, England.

What about dear Anne-Maidlin being born and brought up in East Germany now living in England for the first time? Shocking! She was at first shocked at the visible appearance of everything in, and around Stourbridge and the Waldorf School. Its rather uncared for surroundings and all those male teachers with beards, everything looked so unkempt she thought. Because of these impressions, she became ill with a kidney infection for two or three weeks. However, the very beautiful eurythmy room at the school and our two-eurythmy friends, plus a very friendly faculty helped in our decision to dig in there. In a short time, Anne-Maidlin became the much loved curative eurythmist for the school. Students for the training began coming in toward the end of the summer, and so we began with seven students in our first year! Three teachers were responsible for bringing us to the Stourbridge Waldorf School. One of them lived on the top floor of the main building. When he'd see me go by, he would pop his head out of the upstairs window and say, "Well, Norman, they're piling in!!" (Another phone call) It was a month before we began- and when we advertised six months earlier, we had given his phone number, since we had not our phone yet. So he received the calls from the interested students. "Yes," he said, "They're piling in." Of course seven students is not exactly "a piling in" number, but he was so happy that the school was going to start! He became one of the loving members of our original "council of management," the strongest "heart" person on the committee!

In fact, in the second year of our existence in Stourbridge, he, his wife, Anne-Maidlin and I had a holiday together in France. We drove down in his car. I remember him saying quite seriously – when visiting a particularly interesting village: "Now folks, behave yourselves. Always say 's'il vous plait' and 'merci' and the polite phrases he had taught us. Don't let our country down!!!- Don't look out of place!!" We three had a laugh about his not letting the country down – and he would get rather upset if one of us went into a shop just to look around but didn't buy anything. Oh, yes, he had his foibles, but he was so loving and happy. We couldn't get angry with him! Anne-Maidlin and I lived for the first four years in two rooms in the Waldorf School – with no heat on the weekends, and the smell from the school kitchen just under us, which, when it was onion day, was indescribable! (Raw onions being peeled the night before.)

We were lucky to have Francis Edmunds, the founder of Emerson College in Forest Row, Sussex, as our spiritual leader, so to speak. He gave the first talk to the Stourbridge community at the end of the first year, which included a small presentation from the performing group at that time (four of us). Francis came every year to teach our students about a variety of subjects, such as our bony system, Shakespeare, Parsival, the twelve senses and many other themes. Always about three weeks before he was to come I would call him to remind him of the date. Then he'd ask me what he should talk about. I'd tell him what I thought. He would agree, and then show up at the appointed time. Then came the first lesson with him, and he would say, "Norman said I should talk about (whatever it was) but I will only touch on that theme because I want to take up something else with you." The students would look at me questioningly. I would smile weakly and say, "Go ahead." Now, after three years of this game, when I called him for the usual confirmation of date, again came the question from him, "What do you want me to teach?" I said, "Dear Francis, please do whatever you feel they would need – you do that anyway!" We had a good laugh over that, and for all the following years to come until shortly before his death in November 1989, he was able to inspire our students with his great heart forces, filled with knowledge and humility. One student said, "When Francis is with us, it is like being in church."

And so we lived in the Waldorf School with the raw onion smell streaming up through the floorboards for four years; with no central heating on weekends. Besides the beautiful eurythmy room, we were able to use two barrack-type huts attached to each other, so that from the outside it looked like one long wooden building. (The Waldorf School didn't need them for their classrooms any more.)

In the first two years, once a week, we would arrange "foreign supper menus" in our small kitchen for our students. So, for example, the "Italian supper" meant spaghetti with tomato meat sauce. The "Greek Supper" would be spaghetti with feta cheese and olive oil. The "Indian Supper" would be spaghetti with tandoori or tamari sauce, and the "Mexican

Supper" spaghetti with hot chili peppers. We had great fun with this idea, always spaghetti as the theme. Then, I think in our second year, we were able to buy an old car. The motor ran on large fat rubber bands of some sort! On some weekends we piled five of the students plus we two into the car – some sitting on laps, of course, and drove over the border into Wales, avoiding main roads and the police, because of the over full car. Oh, how wonderful it felt driving into another land, about one and a half hours away from Stourbridge. We stopped for fish and chips – quite an experience for foreign students. In all the seventeen years, we had not more than six or eight English students! Yes, the first four years were like one happy family. At the beginning of each year, Anne-Maidlin gave her talk to the new students on what they were expected to wear in lessons and practices – right down to the underwear! No matter what size of bosom, all were expected to wear bras and petticoats. Anne-Maidlin very often was the inspirer for many of the yearly festivals. Students often were inspired as well. The idea of the Michaelmas tradition of forging with fire, and hammering eurythmy rods, which all the students took part in, with the help and facilities of the woodwork and sculpture teacher, came from Anne-Maidlin.

Then came the time when those old dilapidated huts had to be removed, because an extension was to be built on the same site – a social adventure of great proportions! Firstly, the huts were carefully taken apart piece by piece by professionals, and those bits were piled up in a small field behind the school. There, we teachers and students were to help the professionals re-erect the building with some changes. The neighbors on the other side of the field, and very nearby, objected – and the town council agreed that we just couldn't build there. So, we, the teachers and the students had to move each piece from where it was up to the other side of the school, where there was space and no one could object. It was quite a sight to see seventeen students and four teachers, each gripping a part of a gigantic A-frame (there were four of them), lifting it on signal together, and running it up the short grassy hill on the other side of the field to the new building site! The four A-frames held the roof and walls in place when erected. No, we didn't re-erect the building. This had to be done by professionals. We only helped in small ways, as I said. We were a real community. It was a joy, this togetherness at that time. It took about two and a half months to re-erect the two huts. In the meantime, Elmfield Waldorf School came to the rescue by clearing out two classrooms in the afternoons for our use. This all took place about four years after we started.

Just two years before this adventure, in 1983 one of the Anthroposophical institutions located in Forest Row purchased a house for our use which became our student house. We decided to tear down all the walls dividing up the four bedrooms upstairs, take down the chimney and create a eurythmy practice room. The builder said the work would be "a piece of cake." This house was a five-minute walk to the Waldorf School, and had a large garden which we made good use of! Finally, we didn't need to rent a church room any more (a twenty-minute walk away). But, one early winter morning, when we were still using the church, I was on my way to teach the first lesson there, at 8:15 a.m. It was just getting light, as I started out on my bike. A car turned into the side road on which I was biking. Both car and bike moved towards each other. The car driver didn't see me as he went over the centre line and hit me – all very slow, almost slow motion. I went down with the bike and scraped my leg, (I was more concerned about my bike, but luckily both bike and leg could be repaired). The car driver stopped, very worried. A student from my class who saw it all, told me to go home and rest, while they would practice. But I told her to tell no one. I was going to work! I put some rags around my bleeding leg under my trousers and went on to teach. The leg hurt, but I didn't limp and no one noticed. After the lesson I went to the Waldorf school, where I knew Maidlin was teaching. I made the mistake of calling her out of her curative session and told her the whole story in a very relaxed manner and said I only had a small cut on my leg. I felt alright. She immediately cancelled the rest of her morning lessons, and went home with me, very upset and worried. She gave me some arnica and crataegus pills to take for my heart and shock and then she told me to lie down. When I looked at her, she was pale and almost in shock. So I told her she must take the pills as well! Lie down! That was my dear wife and friend, always more concerned for me than for herself. And I? Well, never mind that now, perhaps later.

Then the day came when our friends, the Joiners with whom we had gone to France, left Elmfield School to start another Waldorf School in Wales. That was in 1985 I believe. Everyone was sad about them leaving, especially ourselves, for they were our staunch supporters! But they felt they were called to go. We bought their house, and finally moved out of the flat at the school. It was the first and only house we were ever to own (my dear mother helped us to buy it). Anne-Maidlin made it a joyful home! Whenever she came into a room, it was like a sunrise! Everyone said this about her! We made some changes in the house, adding a small back and front porch, expanding the size of the kitchen, with skylights in the ceiling. We also had a fireplace installed and the walls of the third floor were finished in wood. Most important of all was the building of a small practice room in what had been our garage. It was needed and became well used. It was all done properly, with a high ceiling, sprung wooden floor and wood panelling covering one third of the way up the walls.

We had occasional "parties" in our small garden and once I played for the students recordings of Glenn Miller, my favorite band when I was a teenager. After two or three selections, I asked them what one could learn from listening to this music for eurythmy. They didn't know, so I said just listen to the joy of togetherness ! They got the point.

After much red tape our training was finally approved of in 1986 by the Section of Performing Arts in Dornach, the center of the Anthroposophical Society; and so we were on our way! Then the Eurythmy School grew, and in 1990/1991 we were with the 28 students in four years, at our pinnacle. Our most glorious moment was the performance of our graduating class doing "The Ancient Mariner" by Coleridge, at the Goetheanum. I told this class of 1991 after they had done a tour of England with their program which featured "The Ancient Mariner," that they should not expect great compliments for their performance in Dornach. They were simply an average class of graduates. The class reacted rather limply and one of them said to me, "Norman, you should be encouraging us, rather than making us feel not good enough!" – Well, maybe so – but I didn't want them (or we teachers for that matter) to be disappointed in the response to our performance. The tour beforehand, in England, which consisted of about 15 performances did not go badly, but as I said, it was not especially outstanding, except for the humour at the end. (That almost always go well, with the unconscious mixture of mime and eurythmy.) So all plans for the safari to Dornach were made. The students rented a mini-bus with room for all the dresses and costumes as well. We three teachers, my wife, a co-worker and myself, were going by plane. So, off we all went, the students leaving one day ahead of us. We planned to meet at a certain time in a certain place in Dornach. On the plane I said to my colleagues, "Shouldn't we make plans to leave Dornach as soon as the performance is over, and have a holiday in the Swiss Alps? That way we'll avoid criticism the following day!" We had all decided earlier, teachers and students, to not run back home but stay in Switzerland for another ten days. Well, we did not make plans to escape and it was fortunate that we didn't. Here is what happened.

We arrived; we all met together and were assigned a 45 minute slot to do a lighting rehearsal and a 45 minute slot to do a dress rehearsal. Our first shock! Most lighting rehearsals for an hour program usually take anywhere from two to three hours, and dress rehearsals, with stops, occasionally one and a half hours. With so many groups performing all within a week, that was the best they could do for each one. (I understand one receives much less time today.) My wife never took part in helping with lighting rehearsals and so it was up to our co-worker and myself, and of course, the lighting engineer. We zipped through each piece, the best we could, when my co-worker suggested a nuance of lighting for one part I almost always said "fine!" – even if I didn't always agree. I think she did the same when I suggested something and so we were able to shoot through the lighting rehearsal in 45 minutes!! At the end of it, the lighting technician came to us, (he was sitting behind us the whole time, changing the lighting as we suggested) and said; "How do you do it? No arguments, both agreeing with each other, this never happens here in Dornach. We always have tensions, arguments, etc., at lighting rehearsals, I take my hat off to you! Is it always like this in England? What a wonderful experience! Thank you so much!" We just looked at each other and smiled meekly. I said, "yes, pretty much." (This was generally true, even without the deadline.)

The dress rehearsal did not go well, and again I thought – we must leave the day after the performance; the Swiss Alps are so beautiful...! This way I won't have to make excuses for the performance, you know, like too tired, strange land, not enough sleep, the little rehearsal time, strange food, etc. All rather half-truths. The big night came: I had to make an introductory speech which I did in English. Anne-Maidlin and our co-worker were behind the stage holding their breath for me and hoping – after telling me what I should say and rehearsing with me weeks before – would I remember it all? (They were behind the stage because they had to help the students with quick dress changes, when necessary, and I was sitting in the audience with the lighting technician to give him cues for each change.)

My wife told me afterwards that my speech seemed to be alright, only at the end of it I was to translate it all into German. So I asked those to please raise their hands who didn't understand the English and if there were some, I would say it in German. No one raised their hand – and I was relieved! We could get started with the programme. I was told after the performance that I had asked the audience in English, if anyone didn't understand the English, I would then say it in German! We were all amused by this and had a good laugh.

So the program was about to begin! A boiling hot evening, with on and off pouring rain, that pelted down on the roof of the building we were in, the wooden building called the Schreinerei (Workhop). The audience was in still expectation as the curtain opened toward the end of the introductory music to set the mood for "The Ancient Mariner." As the piece progressed I could only occasionally look up to see how it was going, since I had to give the lighting cues. Once, I looked up and a saw an unbelievable moment in the movement that chilled my bone marrow. It was just the part where I had tried in vain months earlier to get them to bend their bodies. I saw them bending so beautifully! It had not been there in the practices, or in any of the previous performances. They were together throughout, like never before! Then at a moment in the text where it says, something like … and the rain came down in pouring pelts … just at that moment the rain suddenly did come bucketing down on the roof which one clearly heard! Then at some high dramatic moment later in the text, there was a crack of thunder! Just at the right time enhancing the drama ten-fold. All wonderful, natural, sound effects!

There often were moments in this 30 minute poem, where quick changes of costumes were necessary. My wife and our co-worker, who were behind the curtain in the wings, were there ready holding the next dress, as one or two came flying off the stage, having to be back in 10 or 20 seconds! Well, they were all sweated up from the heat and humidity (which made the dresses stick to their bodies, like glue. The dresses had to be peeled off piece by piece, and the new dress peeled on. It took more time and was always exciting and irritating. "Can we make it on time for the next cue?" (Under normal conditions, the eurythmists can quickly slip on and off the dress by themselves, like water flowing through moss). But the entire programme, the music, the humorous items all went better than at any other time. Our speaker and our musicians did their very best! In short the performance was blessed from above – that was clear. It was the high point of our school which then was balanced by the tragedy which followed eight years later. But, I don't want to get ahead of our story. As the curtain came down to end the program, (I was still thinking about where we could go to hide, to get away from Dornach), there was a stamping of feet and clapping that lasted at least ten minutes! People piled up backstage to congratulate us and the students. Some eurythmists who were not especially friendly to our work suddenly became friendly (and to this day!). My wife and our co-worker, upon hearing the prolonged applause, ran to each other from the opposite sides of the closed curtain – embraced each other, jumping up and down saying, "We did it! We did it!" Just after the performance the lighting engineer asked me if he could keep the lighting notes (the pages where changes of lighting were indicated). These notes have no value after a performance. But he wanted them for a souvenir in remembrance of the strongest working-together of eurythmists he had ever experienced.

I was asked by the students of the Berlin School to meet with them the following day. They encircled me, and told me that they wanted to contribute the money they had received for their performance to our school, to help build our new building, which I had mentioned in my introduction. I tried to refuse because I knew they were themselves in financial difficulties, but they insisted saying that such beautiful work should be supported and that we students and not our teachers can decide what to do with the money.

Obviously we all stayed in Dornach for the next 10 days. We were stopped on the street at least three or four times each day by one person or another who had been in the audience, saying how wonderful it had been! One of the old time experienced eurythmists couldn't believe there were only seven people on stage. She said it seemed to her 15 people at times! It was generally felt that we and the Spring Valley Group were the outstanding contributions that summer. That was not our last contribution to the eurythmy marathon each July, but by far the most impressive.

After this fantastic performance in Dornach in 1991, graced from the heavens, a pianist, who we needed and his eurythmist wife joined our initiative at my invitation. Now, we didn't really need another eurythmist, but they belonged together – so we bought the package – and we all thought what a good combination. They had something to offer a bit different from "our way" – but we all wanted to give it a try. When they came they began working with the students in such a way that actually harmed our way of work which we had built up over thirty years. Well, that was the beginning of the downfall of the Eurythmy School. Tension built up, slowly but surely and after one year we told them they had to leave. It was too confusing for the students – two different ways of working (which could be fruitful after a training) was simply too difficult for the students to digest. The difficulties increased when the pianist started criticizing the way I taught in front of the students. Unfortunately, we were persuaded by a "high standing" community member to try one more year. We did this. We all tried to work together, but it didn't work. After two years we were again persuaded to try again. (I can't to this day, understand why we did not stick to our decision to have them leave – except perhaps, that we wanted to attempt a Michaelic deed, as one of our council member put it, show our good will). Our council would have stood behind us after the two year trial, if we had fired them, but after the third year, it was not possible any more. We, Anne-Maidlin and myself, learned through bitter experience, that it is not possible to work with just anyone who comes along. This nightmare of the last seven years of the school, along with other things, worked to the detriment of Anne-Maidlin's health.

I hasten to add that we had in the 17 years at various intervals of time eight teachers, four of which we really wanted to keep and who really wanted to become part of our faculty. Yet all four had unfortunately to leave for quite personal reasons. Sadness surrounded these partings. Each one was only able to stay between two terms and two years. Could one say, it was in the stars that the school was to close, which it did in 1998? One year before the closure, Anne-Maidlin came to me in the kitchen of our house and said in a pained voice which trembled through her body: "Norman, I think we have to close the school." I'll never forget how she looked as she said it – her body bending slightly sideways, with a heavy, sad voice as if to announce a death in the family – which, in fact it was. A year later the school closed.

Students told us after they graduated that they found our way of teaching very rewarding, harmonizing. They also very much appreciated the fact that we treated them, as far as possible, as friends, listened and tried to include their suggestions, if we found it would not compromise the training process. I suppose one could say that our training was different from the other trainings in as much as we built in therapeutic elements and included these as part of the artistic process. We also included many of the basic eurythmy elements in the work itself and not only as separate exercises but also in the training through out the four to five years. (For those more interested in our work, please refer to the recently published book *Rediscovering the Sources of Eurythmy*, Norman Francis Vogel, with classroom notes by Anne-Maidlin Vogel. Verlag am Goetheanum 2001).

The one ray of light during those last years of the School was the eurythmy research–demonstration study which we began in the last three years before the school closed. This went well, and with five other eurythmists we went twice on mini tours to show very special eurythmical elements which were inspired by Rudolf Steiner's statements in a number of his lectures.

During these last seven years Anne-Maidlin began doing a little less in the eurythmy school, much to the disappointment of the students, but the work went on reasonably well. After this great Dornach success in 1991 she and I were more often separated for short intervals. For me, this was not easy. We never discussed it and we both accepted it. She and I both needed this individual work, as we were otherwise always together. We lived for and with each other day and night, year in and year out. We had our separate conferences to go to for a few days or a week. As time went on, she became more and more involved in curative eurythmy – with children from the Waldorf School, with private patients and with meetings with curative eurythmists in the wider area. I occasionally joined these meetings as I am also a curative eurythmist, but it wasn't really "my thing," as it was hers. I spent more and more time with the students, with graduate student teaching

– even occasionally teaching in different countries. Yet the relationship between us became increasingly strained and although we both knew we belonged together, outer distractions, coming mainly from me, gave her sometimes great sorrow. Yes, we had less time together when we were not doing eurythmy.

Anne-Maidlin spent much more time, in the last 4 to 5 years of the school, with her curative eurythmy responsibilities and as I said less time with the eurythmy school. Nevertheless we still had great walks in the Lakes District and elsewhere. We attended wonderful concerts, and very fine Shakespearean theatre. No one noticed, not even doctors,, that her increased tiredness was the beginning of the coming out of the illness that was in her for many years. It was well covered up by her strong will, eurythmy, joy of life and people, for many, many years. (Two clairvoyants suggested this to me after her passing and this rang true to me). The increasing pain she had to take in those last seven years from co-workers and me made the illness come out and probably led to an earlier death than might have been. Who knows?

During these last seven years, living in the house with her was almost like living alone. She, always, preparing lessons. I wanted so badly to study together with her. She hardly had time for that or when she had time, I did not. She was becoming a fairly well-known curative eurythmist occasionally receiving calls from teachers all over the world, wanting advice about the patients they had.

After the closure of the school she spent some weeks in Park Atwood – an Anthroposophical clinic nearby. A few weeks later we moved to the Filder Klinik, near Stuttgart, where she was treated for eight weeks (July, August 1998). During this time she insisted I should return to England and take her place teaching in the curative eurythmy training in Peredur, East Grinstead. I did this plus my work at this training in the curative tone eurythmy. I called her every day and she was almost always joyful on the telephone. Her doctor thought she would get a little better in time. After the eight weeks at this clinic, I returned to her and we moved together to her doctor brother's sanatorium in Schloss Hamborn, Germany. We had rooms next to each other, and I cared for her along with the doctor and nurses, day and night. I learned how to give injections and massage and took her for walks every day, sometimes in a wheelchair. She was very happy and called me "her best nurse." She did not expect all that love and attention from me. There were nights when her light would go on at two or three in the morning, I would notice this as we had an adjoining balcony. I would get up, go to her door, open it and say "Are you alright?" She would be sitting on the bed and would say "I'm fine, go back to bed." There would be other nights when I woke up and the light would not be on, then I was really frightened, so I would creep to her door, open it quietly, expecting the worst, tip-toeing as close as I could get to her face to try to feel her breathing. As we were almost nose to nose and I still did not feel her breathing, I got very worried. Then in a quiet but strong whisper she would say, "go back to bed, I'm fine." Actually, the last nine months of her life was a time of joy and real happiness between us, it was a wonderful catharsis for the pain and tension of the last seven years.

After seven months in Schloss Hanborn we both moved to her home, in Jena, where she was born and where one brother and one sister lived. She was getting weaker. I had heard about a wonder doctor near Innsbruck who had healing hands. We went there, he saw her everyday and instead of healing she got diarrhoea. This made her even weaker. We were still determined to find our new home in Germany. She had even bought two plates, two cups and two saucers in delightful colors to start our new life together, we thought. After two weeks with this doctor, we drove fourteen hours to Unterlengenhardt, Germany, where there is an anthroposophical clinic. She was exhausted when we arrived. In her diary she wrote "I'm dead tired, I have never been so tired since my illness began." Two days in the clinic was all she had left in this life. She passed over the threshold at 12:35 a.m. on May 21, 1999. On that last night I said to her "Maidlin, you have to fight hard to get through this night." She answered and these were her last words, "Don't worry, Norman, I'll be alright in the morning. It's only another crisis, my soul is perfectly healthy." When she said this, she knew she was dying but wanted me not to worry. All through her life she protected me even with her last breath.

Now, thinking back over the last ten years or so, I can see it could well be that she made herself more busy than she had to, to dull the human disappointments she had with others and with me. Nevertheless I can now also see that she avoided looking at her sadness squarely in the face. And I didn't really see all that, being so self-absorbed. Her disappointment in me came out in her occasionally speaking to me in a disrespectful tone of voice in the last few years. And unfortunately I returned it in a like manner. Yet the work went on beautifully. And it was always a joy, whenever we went on holidays together.

Anne-Maidlin was one of the three leaders of the curative eurythmy training in Peredur, England for 14 years – teaching over 500 students in curative eurythmy in that time. She was loved by all – giving fully to all whom she had contact.

I still to this day (2002) three years after her passing, wonder with deep sadness, and sometimes anger why the spiritual world didn't create a miracle for her, didn't give her more years to live. Why couldn't they wait a while? She was so loved and needed here, and she was in her blossoming time of life. Time in the spiritual world is not so important as here on earth (or so I think), but time on earth is very important. So why couldn't they just wait and give her a chance to deepen her curative work? She once said during her illness, and because of her illness, "Now I know how to work deeper and I want to help very ill people."

Well, that is not what life brought. But I can't help thinking she was cheated. She could have done much more, she had much more to give. This is my personal, admittedly limited picture of this tragedy and is a major sorrow for me. I am aware that there are much wiser Beings at work with a more complete overview covering many incarnations. The head may think this yet the heart still aches.

So now as I live within the memories of our shared life together I am reminded of further telling scenes revealing Anne-Maidlin's being, both in relation to myself as well as in her work with students colleagues and friends.

I think it was in 1994 or 1995 in December, that I had to have an operation- which took place in Herdecke, Germany. (The surgeon who operated on me was an amateur musician and on Christmas day, he, his wife and three children came and gave a little concert for the ward on recorders and flutes, with singing and refreshments, of course.) The night before the operation I was quite worried and a bit frightened. Anne-Maidlin hadn't yet arrived from England. Then suddenly, as I lay in bed trying in vain to fall asleep, a wave of calm came over me, it was so strong, I was somehow reassured that I'd be alright. No, no voices, no seeing of "beings," simply a strong calming feeling filling me completely! In the morning, the calmness was still with me and I was taken to the operating room at 8:15 a.m. (Still no Anne-Maidlin).

The operation went well and I was wheeled back forty-five minutes later. There she was! waiting for me, sorry she had not made it earlier. Oh, how happy we were to see each other! In the next twelve days in the hospital we spent our most beautiful Christmas ever together! (Anne-Maidlin was able to stay in the nearby nurse's quarters). I in bed, she by my side during the day. Now we could finally read to each other every day! And how my dear wife decorated the room with pictures, moss, rocks, figurines and branches! The hospital room was transformed. On the wall facing my bed, was a large painting of Saint Martin and the beggar. (Saint Martin is Anne-Maidlin's birthday saint.)

Anne-Maidlin was now and then giving little presents to the students, our co-workers, to patients, and to me! She often had surprises for everyone. Many years earlier she bought me two very similar looking red winter coats. I said, "Maidlin, why two?" She answered, "One is for Sunday (the slightly better looking one, but very slightly), the other for everyday!" She showed her love for people, for life, for me. She made love visible, here, on earth.

What can I say about our deep inner relationship? She always showed the same love to me – day in, day out – serving me, the eurythmy, her patients and co-workers. She once said to a close friend, "I am on earth to serve," and that she did. Sometimes it was hard for me to tell when she was in suffering, as she almost always succeeded in "pushing away" negative vibrations or soul pain, pushing it all away from herself, not wanting really to look at a difficult situation or at least, not wanting to talk about it. She mostly gave the impression that everything was under control – until the last two or three years of her life – before her illness broke out. I'm afraid, I must confess, I was often responsible for her disappointments in me, which was hard for her to take. My blindness to her needs made her very sad. I was too busy with my own joys and pleasures. Oh yes, the work went on, and actually very well – but that was only one side of the story. From my present view three years after Anne-Maidlin's passing, I feel personal human relationships are still perhaps more important than any "great work" being created. (I have awakened to this only since she has been gone). I missed surrounding her soul with warmth, warmth, warmth, She didn't look like she needed it – and I did not see this need.

With all the disillusionments, plus the very hard path I chose for a life, she followed and never left me. She managed to bring out courage, joy and enthusiasm in all situations. She always made the best of difficult situations, and there were many of them especially in the last seven years. She chose to stand by me on "the path less travelled" as Robert Frost wrote. She chose to stand behind, in front and next to a man who did not belong to the accepted "club" of eurythmists, but went on an individual, deep, meditative way, which she protected and sacrificed much for, and which she firmly believed. She did just that: and she was always by my side, supporting me while she at the same time deepened her curative eurythmy work. How could she do this? – Such strength of will and love!

When Anne-Maidlin and I looked at each other, we often saw the eternal in each other. How difficult it is to live out of our eternal beings in the dance of day-to-day life!

I suppose there have been other marriages with such closeness as ours. But they are certainly rare – very rare! With the Eurythmy School teaching, we never prepared lessons together. It was not necessary – we never discussed what the students should be taught or in what order of development. This was self-understood. Anne-Maidlin knew that I knew how over the four years the tone eurythmy should be developed. I knew that she knew how the speech eurythmy should, step by step, progress over the years. In the work we were like one being coming from entirely different backgrounds! The East and the West met in Vienna. That was karma. Our great teachers, Trude Thetter and Friedl Meangya, representatives of the real middle Europe culture, molded us into one cosmic eurythmic being on Earth.

In the last ten years of our life together I would go to her room at bedtime and say to her "sleep well, Annabelle" and she would answer, as she lay in her bed, "you too, Uncle Lou." That was our signing off for each night.

Some curative eurythmists have told me that since her passing there have been times that they knew they had received help from her during a curative session with a child or adult. One told me that he just did not know what to do with the child he had standing before him. Suddenly he inwardly heard Anne-Maidlin telling him the next exercise for the child.

I feel that the success I am having in the research post-graduate eurythmy work, especially in England and Vienna, is due to her help. She seems to be accompanying me through my final years on earth.

She was, and is the purpose of my life – my nourishment! I feel her presence sometimes more strongly than other times. Her love of humanity, and joy in working with other streams, down to all who knew her to help make us better than we are on earth.

So when I think of our whole life together, I see it was filled with great contrasts. On the one hand, joys, especially in the early days- whilst cooking, eating, hitchhiking all over Europe, theatre-going, concerts and operas. And on the other hand, the slow but sure inner human separation between us, because, especially the last 15 years, Anne-Maidlin took leaping steps forward year by year in the inner social realm. She learned to really understand the people who sometimes criticized me, and occasionally even her. I was not able to follow her ever deepening humanity, and so I was frustrated, jealous at times of her popularity, and simply remained blind to her needs, which I must say she kept well hidden from me. She would say nothing: just she waited for me to take a step in freedom in the direction of "Community Building" – a step I was not able to take – didn't even know how to try. When she said to me, "If you could only become friends with him!" (one who criticized me and my work sharply). I said, "I just couldn't do it." (I was too weak). She said, after some days, " Yes, Norman, I see you can't, I understand."

There never was any serious thought of leaving each other. She sacrificed her life for me! That's the cross I have to bear now in this life this time! A heavy burden. I often ask myself the question: "Did Maidlin die of cancer or of a broken heart?"

If I am able to take into my being sincerely, reverently, humbly, the Being of Christ, we will be able to meet each other consciously after I pass over. And yet, with all the pain she had she could write for my birthday in 1994:

To my belovest Norman!

Now the Door to wisdom opened wide
Hassels, unimportance lay aside
Let the Light from yonder side
shine trough
And illumen your real inner You!

I will allway's walk close to your side
Hand in Hand, we for the Truth will stride!

Sept. 7, 1994
with all my Love
your Maidlin.

www.ingramcontent.com/pod-product-compliance
Lightning Source LLC
Chambersburg PA
CBHW080811280326
41926CB00091B/4252